THE MATCH

The Match

"Savior Siblings" and
One Family's Battle to
Heal Their Daughter

Beth Whitehouse

BEACON PRESS
BOSTON

Beacon Press
25 Beacon Street
Boston, Massachusetts 02108-2892
www.beacon.org

Beacon Press books
are published under the auspices of
the Unitarian Universalist Association of Congregations.

13 12 11 10   8 7 6 5 4 3 2 1

This book is printed on acid-free paper that meets the uncoated paper ANSI/
NISO specifications for permanence as revised in 1992.

Text design by M. F. Rutherglen
at Wilsted & Taylor Publishing Services

Portions of this book are based upon a series of articles by
Beth Whitehouse, which appeared in *Newsday* in 2007.
The author gratefully acknowledges permission from
Newsday to reprint those sections.

The excerpt from the essay "Life Saver," from *Teen Vogue*, appeared
in the February 2009 issue. It is reprinted here with permission.
Copyright © 2009 Condé Nast Publications. All rights reserved.

Library of Congress Cataloging-in-Publication Data

Whitehouse, Beth.
The match : "savior siblings" and one family's battle to heal their daughter /
Beth Whitehouse.
p. cm.
ISBN 978-0-8070-7286-8 (hardcover : alk. paper)
1. Trebing, Katie—Health. 2. Anemia in children—Patients—New York (State)—New
York—Biography. 3. Bone marrow—Transplantation—Patients—New York (State)—
New York—Biography. 4. Pure red cell aplasia—Patients—New York (State)—New
York—Biography. 5. Fertilization in vitro, human. 6. Procurement of organs,
tissues, etc. I. Title.

RJ416.A6T74 2010
362.198'921520092—dc22   2009035949

For my grandmother Bobbie,
who always wanted me
to write a book;

For Sandra and Don Whitehouse,
my mom and dad,
who gave me the nature and
nurture to be able to do so;

And for my son, Tristan,
who made me understand why
parents would do anything
to help their children

CONTENTS

PRELUDE

Stacy Trebing yanked off the yellow paper hospital gown that covered her shorts and T-shirt, unhooked the surgical mask from behind her ears, and stuffed both items into the garbage pail in the entryway of her daughter's hospital room. She'd been at her three-year-old daughter's bedside practically every minute of the past ten days.

She needed a breather.

The next morning, Stacy's daughter would have a bone marrow transplant, a medical procedure that would either cure her or kill her. Every minute since Katie's birth had been leading to this day. Everything Stacy and her husband, Steve, had done, every decision they'd made, had propelled them here.

Including the most controversial of their choices: to create a new human being they had selected as an embryo because he genetically matched a critical portion of his sister's DNA.

That one-year-old baby would be brought into the hospital the following morning to donate the life-changing bone marrow that was the only chance to heal his sister. Christopher Trebing was born to be a member of the Trebing family, but he was also born with a job to do. He would be put under general anesthesia while a doctor inserted needles repeatedly into his hips and siphoned the tissue that could repair Katie's ailing body.

Stacy headed to the ninth floor's family sitting room at Memorial Sloan-Kettering Cancer Center in Manhattan and sank onto the couch. It had been an exhausting time readying Katie's body for the transplant, watching chemotherapy drugs flow like poison into her daughter's body, knocking out Katie's immune system so her body couldn't fight off Christopher's gift.

Katie seemed so different from her usual spirited self. Just one month earlier, she had been bouncing on the trampoline in the Trebings' backyard, her white poncho flying into the air as she ricocheted up and down. Katie, who loved to race to the basement and dart back upstairs dressed in her pink fairy costume with wings. Katie, whose dimples were cut into her cheeks as though they'd been etched with diamonds.

But now Katie had zero immunity to any foreign invader, no defense against any germs, and a common cold could mean tragedy. She was in isolation in a hospital room, attached to a web of IV tubes.

Katie and Christopher wouldn't see each other on what the doctors called Day Zero. Katie would stay in isolation in her room, and Christopher's marrow would be transported in an IV bag and dripped into her. Doctors told Stacy that because it had been so difficult to get an IV into Christopher's veins during his preoperative blood testing, they might have to go through a more dangerous route, a vein in his leg, to administer anesthesia. Stacy feared for both children.

As she sat, Stacy wasn't dwelling on the many ethical issues that troubled the bioethicists and critics who thought no baby should be conceived with a purpose: Who would protect the medical interests of what was referred to as a "savior sibling" when his parents were so focused on curing the older child? How would such a baby feel when he grew up and learned he had been brought into the family with a responsibility? Who would object if the child was later called upon to donate something more radical than bone marrow to help the sibling—a kidney perhaps?

As his mom, Stacy had more personal concerns: How would she feel if Christopher's much-anticipated bone marrow donation didn't work? What if Katie's body rejected Christopher's marrow and Katie died? Would it change how Stacy felt about Christopher? Would it make it hard to be his mother? *If anything ever happened to Katie,* Stacy asked herself uneasily, *would I be resentful toward him?*

1

"Mind If I Take One Last Ski Run?"

Snowflakes fell lightly onto Stacy Olsen as she rang Jane Ann Mc-Bride's doorbell. Inside the house on Long Island, the McBride family's annual Christmas party was in full swing. Steve Trebing was enjoying a beer, and he glanced at the door as Jane Ann opened it.

As Steve saw Stacy walk inside, things seemed to move in slow motion. Mesmerized, he tried not to stare as Stacy slid her arms out of her jacket and shook it off, then brushed the snowflakes from her short brown hair.

For months, Jane Ann had been trying to play Cupid. She'd grown up with Steve running around with her younger brother, Pete, the boys riding bicycles through their working-class neighborhood and building forts in the patches of nearby woods. Jane Ann had met Stacy at the State University of New York at Stony Brook, where they both were studying to become physical therapists. Jane Ann had repeatedly insisted that Steve should date Stacy, that she was the one for him.

At that moment, Steve believed her.

By the time Steve and Stacy were sharing a cup of tea in the McBrides' kitchen that December night in 1993, Steve had asked Stacy out to dinner, and she'd said yes. The guests had previously planned to spend the night at the McBrides' so they could enjoy cocktails without worrying about driving home safely. When all the chatting ended, Steve found a spot on a couch, took off his glasses, and closed his eyes.

Soon he felt a tug on his arm. Steve was afraid it was Pete or one of his other grade-school buddies waking him up to make him the victim of a sophomoric prank, and he opened his eyes cautiously. To his surprise, Stacy was looking up at him. She'd set up her blankets on the floor next to his couch. Steve shocked himself by reaching down and caressing Stacy's face. Then the two kissed.

With that kiss—what Steve calls "that extraordinary kiss"— began the story of the Trebing family.

On a ski trip with friends to New Jersey's Vernon Valley Great Gorge five weeks into their relationship, Steve knew he was in love. Stacy had just finished blow-drying and styling her hair. "Mind if I take one last ski run before dinner?" Steve asked, fully expecting his new girlfriend to object. Stacy paused, then said, "I'll race you." By the time the two had sashayed to the bottom of that mountain, Steve was hooked.

The following Christmas, Steve, a skinny twenty-three-year-old with black, wavy hair and glasses, found himself knocking on the door of Stacy's parents' house, a bottle of champagne in his hands, wondering if Stacy's parents would agree to let him marry their daughter. Steve had driven past the house three times in his Toyota Tercel before he worked up the courage to go in. "You better have money in your bank account and let her keep her maiden name if she wishes," Pam Olsen told Steve.

That New Year's Eve, on another ski trip, in an après-ski pub in Vermont, Steve schemed with the band. In the midst of a set, band members stopped playing, started a soft drumroll, and called Steve to the stage. He climbed three steps to reach them and took the proffered microphone with a shaking hand.

"First I'd like to wish everyone a healthy and happy 1995," Steve said. Then he asked Stacy to join him on stage. Stacy's best friend,

Maureen Levitan, gave her a push, and Stacy walked to the stage. Steve got down on one knee. "Stacy, will you marry me?" he asked.

Once again, Stacy said yes, with tears in her eyes.

Stacy's parents lived adjacent to the Olsen family nursery in Nesconset, Long Island, about a ninety-minute drive east from Manhattan. Stacy's maternal grandparents had moved to the area in the 1950s. Through the years, they purchased surrounding properties. The amount of land they owned grew large enough to accommodate houses for their children and their children's children. Stacy was the youngest by at least ten years of Calvin and Pam Olsen's four children. Her parents, grandparents, two older sisters, and older brother all eventually had houses on the same two blocks. It was like the Kennedy compound.

For a while after Steve and Stacy married, they lived in an apartment above the nursery that Stacy's sister Leslie ran. Stacy worked as a physical therapist. Steve, who had graduated with a degree in business from the State University of New York at Oswego, bought and ran a flower shop. Steve also began offering party-tent rentals at the florist's shop, and he soon found the tent business more lucrative than the flowers. The stressful flower holidays—Mother's Day, Thanksgiving, Christmas—became a thing of the past as he sold the florist shop and started a business devoted solely to putting up high-end party tents for occasions such as weddings and graduations. Steve's new busy season was June through September; he put up cavernous, white-peaked tents for weddings at vineyards on Long Island's North Fork and at political fund-raisers in the chichi Hamptons. He landed an account to put up tents for the New York City Marathon each November. After a few years, Steve's business was flourishing; Steve juggled dozens of events each weekend, and his warehouse was filled with hundreds of tents. Because they paid little rent, Steve and Stacy used their disposable income to travel to Europe, the Caribbean, and Hawaii. They saved for a house. Life was carefree.

In March of 2000, Steve and Stacy had a son. They named him after Stacy's father, Calvin. Throughout her pregnancy, Stacy sensed she was having a boy because Calvin was so active in the womb. When Calvin was born, Stacy and Steve thought their first child was nothing short of perfect.

The following year, the young Trebings permanently joined the compound, building their dream home on a plot of land next door to Stacy's parents and across the street from her brother, Craig, and her sister Lisa. Stacy's sister Leslie lived one block over, next to Stacy's grandparents' home. Steve and Stacy built a spacious two-story Victorian with a full finished basement, a home far grander than they could have afforded if the land hadn't been a gift.

After Calvin was born, Stacy quit her job to stay home with him. Stacy's kitchen table became family central. The sisters were in and out of one another's homes, coming over to talk about their children, husbands, and responsibilities. Leslie had three daughters; Lisa had a daughter and three stepsons. The women took turns discussing the challenges of parenthood.

Time went so quickly that Steve often felt he didn't even have the chance to cross the days off the calendar. Then, when Calvin was two years old, Stacy got pregnant and gave birth to the Trebings' second child. Their comfortable suburban life suddenly shattered.

Within hours of Kathleen Patricia Trebing's birth, on December 12, 2002, her parents' joy turned to anxiety.

Everything about the delivery at St. Catherine of Siena Medical Center in Smithtown, Long Island, had been normal. Steve was convinced he was about to have another son and was surprised when the obstetrician said the baby was a girl. Stacy, however, had been insisting her whole pregnancy that she'd be giving birth to a daughter. The Trebings named Katie after Steve's and Stacy's mothers. The doctor immediately handed Katie to Stacy, and Katie eagerly breast-fed. Stacy thought Katie looked beautiful.

After the 7:30 a.m. delivery, an ecstatic Steve went home to tell

Calvin he had a sister. Stacy settled into her hospital room to rest before family and friends arrived to meet the newest Trebing.

Then worry arrived with a nurse.

"Katie's blood tests are abnormal," she said. Specifically, the baby's hemoglobin was low. This meant she was not getting enough oxygen in her bloodstream. Now, in the nursery, Katie lay under an oxygen hood, her chest heaving as she labored to breathe.

Stacy called Steve and told him to please rush back. Rattled, Steve arrived in the hospital room just as the doctor said, "There's a problem. We want to make sure it's not her heart." Katie needed to be moved immediately to the neonatal intensive care unit at the regional Stony Brook University Medical Center. Stacy broke down and cried.

"You have to discharge me, because I'm going with her," Stacy insisted. Stacy and Katie left in separate ambulances; Steve drove with Stacy's dad. The neonatal intensive care unit was frightening. Beeping machines. Tubes and wires everywhere. Nurses and doctors bustling through. The Trebings sat elbow to elbow with other parents holding vigil beside bassinets in the NICU, or, as parents who spend a lot of time in the unit call it, the Nick U.

Doctors quickly ruled out a heart problem. But Katie's hemoglobin, the pigment in red blood cells that carries oxygen, continued to plunge. When hemoglobin levels drop, the heart has to pump harder to circulate enough oxygen through the body. That causes stress on even a healthy heart. Katie's doctors wondered whether the obstetrician might have lifted Katie from Stacy's body too quickly, which could have sent too much of Katie's blood back into the umbilical cord. Maybe that explained her problem. To fight the dropping hemoglobin count, Katie needed more blood. So on her first day on Earth, before she knew what it was like to see the moon, Katie had her first blood transfusion.

Steve felt as though he'd been beamed into a television medical drama. Every time he asked the doctors what they thought was wrong, they would say, "We're doing tests." He pushed away fleeting thoughts that his daughter was in mortal danger and tried not to lose control of his emotions. For her part, Stacy, who usually was calmer than Steve in a crisis, saw something promising: Katie was bigger than all the other babies in the unit. They seemed tiny, as many of them were premature, while Katie weighed eight pounds, eleven ounces, the biggest baby there.

Stacy was admitted to Stony Brook as well, since she had given birth only hours before. Though she was physically exhausted, Stacy felt an unusual sense of strength. She felt elated over having a daughter. She couldn't fathom anything being seriously wrong with her baby girl. As she nonetheless tamped down fear, Stacy made a promise to her newborn, and over the next four and a half years, through all the hospital and doctor visits, this promise would become Stacy's mantra, Stacy's prayer: "Everything will be fine."

After that blood transfusion, Katie immediately improved. However, Katie did develop pneumonia because she had inhaled meconium during the birth process. Meconium is a newborn's first stool; sometimes it can be released into the amniotic fluid and accidentally inhaled or swallowed during the delivery. Katie had to stay in the NICU for eleven days and was on antibiotics for twelve days. But otherwise, everything seemed okay. Stacy was discharged from the hospital after a couple of days, but she returned to the NICU at eight o'clock every morning for Katie's first breast-feeding and stayed until early evening. The unit had a rocking chair, and Stacy would hold Katie for hours, bonding with her new baby. Katie had a shock of black hair, and her eyes opened so wide that they seemed to take up most of her face. The days were long. Stacy was still physically recovering from giving birth, and she felt guilty leaving two-year-old Calvin all day. Stacy got home at six in the evening to spend time with Calvin, and she pumped her breast milk every three hours so there'd be enough to leave at the hospital for the nurses to feed Katie overnight. Luckily it was December, a slow season for Steve. He was able to take over the primary daytime responsibility for Calvin. As Stacy and Steve spoke with other parents in the NICU whose babies had been there for months, they realized that in the scheme of things, their situation wasn't so terrible.

Katie came home to Nesconset on December 23, just in time for Christmas. Steve thought his new daughter's discharge seemed like a Christmas present. Katie came home with an oxygen saturation monitor with a clip that the Trebings were supposed to attach to her toe to measure her levels as she slept. But Katie never had trouble breathing again, and the sensor kept falling off her toe and making the alarm go off, so the doctors agreed the Trebings could discontinue the monitor and relax.

That relaxation was short-lived.

2

"What Do You Think It Is?"

Stacy, Katie, and Calvin began to craft a normal routine at home. Stacy took Katie to the pediatrician for a follow-up visit, and she seemed to be thriving. Then in early January of 2003, a couple of weeks after Katie came home from the hospital, a home-health-care nurse made a routine follow-up visit to the Trebing house, a standard procedure for babies who had been discharged from the neonatal intensive care unit. "Did you take Katie for a follow-up blood test?" the nurse casually asked Stacy.

"No," Stacy said, puzzled. "Why?"

The nurse pointed to Katie's discharge papers from Stony Brook University Medical Center. A scribbled note from the doctor read: *Suggest follow-up CBC*. The acronym *CBC* stood for *complete blood count*. Stacy hadn't even noticed it.

The next day, Stacy took Katie back to her pediatrician, Keith Ancona, who sent them to get Katie's blood drawn at the laboratory covered by her insurance. Stacy sat in the waiting room there, fearful that her newborn was being exposed to all the germs of the strangers also waiting to get their blood tested. When Stacy was called in and saw the look on the technician's face, she knew the blood test wasn't going to be easy. The technicians weren't used to drawing blood from newborns; Katie was so tiny they feared they wouldn't be able to find a vein. The lab manager did it. It was the first of what would become weekly blood tests.

After one of those tests a few weeks later, in early February, Dr. Ancona called while Stacy was preparing dinner and Calvin was scampering underfoot. Stacy answered the cordless phone. "You have to take Katie to Stony Brook immediately," Ancona said. A normal hemoglobin count for a child Katie's age measures between 12 and 16; Katie's had dropped to 5. She needed a second blood transfusion right away. Stacy's hope that the transfusion after Katie's birth had fixed whatever was wrong crumpled.

Stacy's mind flashed back to the previous disheartening experience with Katie in the NICU. "Do I really have to?" she asked, already crying.

"She could go into cardiac arrest," Ancona warned. When Steve, Stacy, and Katie arrived at Stony Brook University Medical Center, Katie was admitted to the pediatric unit. She was placed in a crib; Stacy thought her baby seemed so tiny and helpless in there. Katie got her second blood transfusion, and Stacy stayed overnight next to Katie on a recliner, spending sleepless hours wondering what was happening to her daughter.

The hematologist who saw Katie at Stony Brook hoped that during Stacy's pregnancy she had been exposed to parvovirus B19, the virus that causes the usually benign fifth disease. The virus can cause a baby to be born with severe anemia but normalcy eventually kicks in. The doctors started Katie on a drug called Epogen to assist her bone marrow in producing red blood cells. Stacy was sent home and instructed to give her two-month-old baby a shot in the leg every day.

Steve and Stacy did as the doctors instructed. Katie was an unusually alert baby, her eyes following Calvin around and watching Mom and Dad in the living room. Stacy thought she looked just like Stacy's mom had in her infant pictures. When Katie did close her eyes, Steve loved to have her fall asleep in the crook of his arm as he lounged on the couch. Stacy filled in information on Katie's first few months in her "Baby's First Year" book, which had spaces for the first time the baby rolled over and sat up.

But after four weeks of Epogen, Katie's hemoglobin was still too low.

Now that her hemoglobin count was a recurring problem, Katie began regular visits to the hospital as doctors tried to figure out what was wrong. In the back of his mind, Richard Ancona, the father and medical partner of Keith Ancona, suspected a rare disorder. But until he was sure, he didn't want to alarm the Trebings. When Stacy asked, "What do you think it is?" he would reply, "I'm not telling you, because I don't want you to go on the Internet and become a lunatic." What Ancona didn't want the Trebings to find out was that if his suspicion was right, Katie would likely be tied to doctors and hospitals for the rest of her life. At each appointment, Stacy pressured the doctors to tell her their worst fears. Finally, at one of Katie's weekly visits to the Anconas' cheery office with the tennis rackets and baseballs on the borders of the examination room, the doctors gave in. Both Anconas, father and son, entered the exam room and closed the door behind them. Stacy held Katie close, tempted to run. She knew instinctively that something very bad was about to be said. Richard and Keith Ancona spoke softly and carefully as they explained that they thought Katie might have Diamond Blackfan anemia.

That day was the first time Stacy heard the term. The disease, commonly referred to as DBA, was first documented in 1938 by two doctors at Children's Hospital Boston, Louis Diamond and Kenneth Blackfan. It is so rare that probably fewer than a thousand people in North America have it at any point in time. Approximately thirty children are born with this disease each year in the United States and Canada. It affects boys and girls equally and is commonly diagnosed during a child's first year. In a number of cases it is passed on genetically from a parent who carries the mutation; in some cases, it is a new mutation.

This type of anemia is often not recognized immediately because it is so rare. It was a coincidence that the senior Dr. Ancona happened to be a pediatrician who specialized in hematology, diseases of the blood. That's why he'd thought of DBA so early on. Every month, he told Stacy, Katie would need a blood transfusion to supply her with someone else's red blood cells—or she would die.

As Stacy listened in disbelief, she felt the room swirling around her. She tried to understand what the doctors were saying. Keith Ancona put his arm around Stacy; he could see her legs were buckling. Stacy could barely talk through the lump in her throat as she asked the Anconas if she could call Steve and have him come over so they could explain this to him as well.

By the time Steve arrived, Stacy's eyes were red and her cheeks were wet. She tried to fill Steve in before the doctors came back, but she tripped over the medical jargon, and she could see that she was frustrating Steve.

Both Anconas returned to the small exam room, where the four adults and Katie took up most of the space. The senior Ancona took the lead and maneuvered his way to the white-papered exam table. He ripped a fresh sheet of the thin white paper from the roll, took a black marker from his pocket, and began to draw red blood cells. He explained in layperson's terms how they worked, or, in Katie's case, how they didn't. In a normal human body, oxygen is brought into the lungs with each breath. Red blood cells, which are constantly produced in the bone marrow, pick up the oxygen in the lungs and deliver it to the body. Oxygen nourishes tissues and organs throughout the body, allowing it to work efficiently and grow normally. The heart is the pump that keeps all the elements moving along. When a person has DBA, the bone marrow cannot make enough red blood cells to deliver the needed oxygen to the body, and the heart beats harder and faster to compensate. Katie's bone marrow would never make enough red blood cells.

Steve felt heartbroken. He feared for his little girl's future, worried about her treatments, her limitations. It was one of the most overwhelming moments in Steve's life.

Steve and Stacy went home and put Calvin and Katie to bed, then headed to the basement for what would become their routine: reviewing all the information they'd been given that day and trying to help each other make sense of it.

To confirm the Anconas' suspicions, Katie needed a bone marrow biopsy. The definitive answer came in March, when Katie was three months old. Katie returned to Stony Brook University Medical Center for a third blood transfusion, and doctors removed a piece of bone from Katie's hip. That biopsy confirmed Richard Ancona's fear.

On the same day, Steve's mother came to the hospital to donate blood for Katie's next transfusion, something that turned out to be one of the biggest mistakes the Trebings made in Katie's medical care.

In a stroke of good fortune for the Trebings, the doctor who managed the Diamond Blackfan Anemia Registry of North America was based at Schneider Children's Hospital in New Hyde Park, a community on Long Island about an hour from the Trebings' home. The Trebings signed up Katie as a patient of Dr. Jeffrey Lipton, the chief of pediatric hematology/oncology and stem cell transplantation at Schneider Children's Hospital.

When they first went to see Lipton, the Trebings boiled down all of their questions to one: how do we beat this?

Two options treat the disease, Lipton told the Trebings at their first appointment, which lasted for hours: monthly blood transfusions or oral steroids. Katie had already started blood transfusions. Lipton told the Trebings these transfusions would eventually cause iron buildup in Katie's organs. Month after month, year after year, iron would accumulate in the liver and heart, causing the organs to deteriorate.

To combat iron buildup, within twenty-four months Katie would have to be hooked up five nights a week to a pump that would release a drug called Desferal into her system as she slept. The pump would be connected to her body by a needle inserted into Katie's thigh or abdomen. The drug would bind to the iron in Katie's body, a process called chelation, and the bound iron would be eliminated when Katie urinated. She would have to use the drug for the rest of her life, or until scientists came up with a better alternative. The older children got, the more they disliked the Desferal pump and the less likely they were to use it regularly. The needle caused leg pain and itching. Scientists had recently developed a dissolvable oral tablet that might make hooking up to a Desferal pump overnight unnecessary, but no quantity of drugs was guaranteed to rid the body of all excess iron, Lipton explained. "Neither method is perfect," he said.

The monthly transfusions coupled with Desferal only served to keep the DBA under control and put off the inevitable. Current studies showed that more than 40 percent of Diamond Blackfan patients who had to undergo transfusions regularly—referred to as "transfusion dependent"—died by their forties, Lipton said; their organs were worn down and eventually wiped out by the toll of the excess iron.

The second option, oral steroids, could trigger the body's ability to produce red blood cells, but because the steroids also inhibited growth, Lipton wouldn't try it until Katie was at least a year old. (These were corticosteroids, different from anabolic steroids, which is what people sometimes take to increase muscle mass.)

Only about 20 percent of Diamond Blackfan patients went into extended remission without needing any further steroid or transfusion treatment. Moreover, how long such a remission might last was anyone's guess.

About 40 percent of patients could be maintained on an acceptable steady dose of steroids and avoid the need for transfusions. But even if Katie turned out to be what doctors called a "steroid responder," taking steroids had long-term side effects that could include weight gain, high blood pressure, increased susceptibility to infection, glaucoma, cataracts, severe mood swings, and premature osteoporosis, or weakening of her bones. Some patients on long-term steroids have needed joint replacement surgery as early as their twenties. *Each method—transfusions or steroids—is terrible,* Steve thought. Each would have an impact on Katie's longevity, quality of life, and susceptibility to other diseases.

Wasn't there any chance of a cure? Steve and Stacy implored.

Just one, Lipton told them. The only known cure for DBA was a bone marrow transplant from a sibling who had exactly the same human leukocyte antigens (HLA) as the patient.

In effect, these antigens are the code that tells the body's immune system not to attack. Every cell in a human body has a DNA code on it that identifies the cell as a member of the club, so to speak. If another cell appears in the body that does not bear this identical pattern, the immune system treats it as a foreign invader and attacks. That's why bone marrow transplants that use exact human leukocyte antigen matches are the most successful.

In a patient who had a fatal disease, a transplant from a matched stranger culled from the nation's volunteer bone marrow donor registry could be performed. But because DBA was not immediately deadly—though it shortened life span, wreaked havoc on the patient's quality of life, and put the patient at increased risk for developing cancers such as leukemia—doctors didn't normally do this. Transplanting bone marrow from a donor who wasn't a sibling led to a significantly higher risk of death for the patient because of the higher likelihood of rejection. So in DBA, the risks of a bone marrow transplant from someone other than a sibling outweighed the benefits.

Lipton warned the Trebings not to allow family members to donate blood for Katie's transfusions because it could complicate any future bone marrow transplant from a matched sibling, increasing the danger to Katie. Stacy was chagrined that they'd already had Steve's mother donate blood, which they'd used for Katie most recent transfusion, but it was too late to dwell on that error now.

The Trebings were thrilled that they had some possibility of a cure to cling to. They had Calvin tested immediately. If he was a match, they would be able to use his bone marrow to heal Katie.

He wasn't.

The Trebings thought that was the end of hope.

But Dr. Lipton had one more idea.

On the cutting edge of genetics and medicine, where science offered hope to frightened parents of ill children, there was a possible way to provide Katie with a perfect sibling match, Dr. Lipton told the Trebings: have another baby.

The conception of this new baby could not be left to chance, though; the natural odds were that only one in every four of the Trebings' offspring would be an exact match for Katie. Stacy and Steve would have to undergo in vitro fertilization, or IVF, to produce numerous embryos to choose from—sometimes up to twenty from one cycle—to increase the odds of finding a match. Then there would be another step: when the embryos were three days old and still in the laboratory, scientists would pull one cell off of each and use a test called preimplantation genetic diagnosis—commonly referred to as PGD—to find that perfect match. Only those embryos that matched would be implanted in Stacy's uterus.

This baby would be a donor sibling, or, to some, a savior sibling. The umbilical-cord blood would be saved. At the appropriate time, the cord blood would be transplanted into Katie to produce new, healthy bone marrow.

Umbilical-cord blood contains stem cells, which have the ability to rebuild the blood and immune system. After a child's birth, the cord blood can be saved and used in matched siblings to treat diseases such as leukemia and blood disorders such as Diamond Blackfan anemia. When the stem cells are transplanted, they migrate to the malfunctioning bone marrow sites and begin producing bone marrow correctly. In Katie's case, that meant she would be making her own red blood cells on a permanent basis.

In the best-case scenario, the donor child wouldn't be called upon again. However, Lipton warned, if the cord blood wasn't sufficient—if enough couldn't be collected at birth, for instance—the new baby's bone marrow would have to be removed from the hips and transplanted into the patient, a potentially painful procedure for the new child that had to be performed in an operating room under general anesthesia. The Trebings needed to consider whether they were willing to take that path, which involved some medical risk to the new child, including the possibility of an adverse reaction to the anesthesia as well as postprocedure infections.

Whether the transplant was done with the umbilical-cord blood or the baby's bone marrow, it would be a perilous procedure for Katie. She would be isolated in a hospital room for at least a month while doctors used chemotherapy drugs to purposely disable her immune system so that it would be less likely to attack the donor's bone marrow. This step was necessary even with an exact-match sibling. Katie would therefore be susceptible to disease for months; even a common cold could kill her. She'd be isolated even after returning home from the hospital; she'd have to take immune-suppressing drugs for almost a year. In the long run, the chemotherapy might cause premature menopause, and she'd probably never have her own biological children. The transplant gave her a greater than 90 percent chance of being cured, but if the process failed—if Katie got a virus or an infection, or if her body rejected the marrow or vice versa—she could die.

The stacking of the three procedures—fertilization (creating embryos in the lab), diagnosis (testing the embryos in order to select those that matched perfectly), and eventual bone marrow transplant—had first been documented only three years earlier, when a Denver boy named Adam Nash was conceived as a match for his then six-year-old sister, Molly. Molly had a more dangerous bone marrow failure syndrome than Katie—Fanconi anemia—and was close to death at the time of her transplant. Her match, Adam, was born in 2000.

As with many new reproductive technologies, Lipton warned the Trebings, moral, ethical, and medical questions abounded—for families and for society. "It's easy to say someone donated bone marrow or a kidney to a sibling and generally feels pretty good about themselves. But some people think it gets a little presumptuous to say, 'You should be born for this purpose,'" Lipton said.

Steve thought the whole concept was mind-blowing, like something out of science fiction. Steve and Stacy thought about it for months. Stacy called Reproductive Specialists of New York, the local fertility practice that Lipton recommended, and talked to a reproductive endocrinologist named Dr. James Stelling who could perform the in vitro fertilization that would be followed by preimplantation genetic diagnosis. The quest wouldn't guarantee Stacy a pregnancy, Stelling warned her. Just like any other woman who went through IVF, Stacy might not become pregnant on the first try, the second try, or any of her attempts. She would be rolling the dice. But the facts that she and Steve were both in their early thirties and that Stacy was obviously fertile would be in the Trebings' favor.

The Trebings and their extended family members spent a number of nights at their kitchen table talking about what they should do. "I'm glad I'm not you, that I don't have to make this decision, but I'll support any decision you make," Stacy's sister Lisa Holewinski said repeatedly.

While Steve and Stacy were making up their minds, Katie continued to need medical attention.

3

"Never in a Million Years"

Katie's lips were trembling so much her binky was in danger of tumbling from her mouth. Her brown pigtails bobbed as she squirmed in Stacy's lap, first struggling to escape, then melting backward into her mother's chest. A nurse held Katie's arm straight as she tied a thick blue rubber band around Katie's upper arm. She prepped the area with an alcohol pad. Katie watched carefully. Katie was too young for bravery. She was now eighteen months old and on her twentieth blood transfusion. She was afraid of the pinch that she knew was coming. She had a name for it: her boo-boo.

"Let's sing 'Barbara Ann,'" Stacy suggested to the two nurses who stood on either side of Katie in the pediatric hematology unit at Stony Brook University Medical Center. They began to warble the Beach Boys classic. As the singing distracted Katie, nurse Pattie Losquadro—whom Stacy had gratefully nicknamed "One-Shot Pattie"—inserted a needle into the crook of Katie's right elbow. "All done, all done," Stacy whispered to Katie. Katie quickly settled down; she knew the worst part was over.

"When she was first diagnosed I was 'Seven-Shot Pattie,'" Losquadro joked. But Katie and Losquadro had gotten used to each other, and Katie had grown older. That made it easier for Losquadro to glide the needle in. Losquadro taped Katie's right arm to a board and removed the needle, leaving an IV tube in the vein. "We've got you looking like a mummy here," Losquadro said. Katie's brown eyes were still watering.

"We have a new pouty face," Stacy said.

Katie cheered up quickly. On this muggy June day, when thunderstorms were threatening, Katie settled down to spend most of the day in the hospital. With the dreaded needlestick boo-boo behind her, Katie smiled, dimples digging deep into her cheeks. After so many visits, Katie had mastered the secrets of the unit designed for sick children. She wriggled off Stacy's lap and walked to a gray metal file cabinet. No file folders in there. Katie pulled open the second drawer from the bottom, where she knew there was a cache of Cheetos, Three Musketeers bars, Reese's peanut butter cups, and various other treats. Katie chose a miniature chocolate bell wrapped in gold foil and climbed into her stroller to eat it. Soon chocolate was smeared all over her hands and cheeks. She grabbed a hospital curtain with pastel sea horses swimming on it and tried to use it as a napkin. The curtains matched the decor of the pediatric hematology area, where a ribbon in the colors of the rainbow was painted on the wall, and dolphins frolicked outside the department's entryway.

Katie's intravenous line was hooked to a rolling stand with a suspended bag of blood that was pumped into her body over several hours. Stacy's challenge was to keep her daughter—who got more and more energetic as the new blood revitalized her—entertained. They played hide-and-seek with the nurses, Katie too young to realize that her rolling IV stand was a giveaway. There was a box attached to the IV pole that measured the rate of blood flowing in, and sometimes Stacy sat Katie on the box, one leg on each side of the pole, and pushed her around the hematology unit as if the IV stand were a go-cart. They wandered the hallways, counting the fish in the colorful pictures on the walls. Nurse Losquadro brought out a gymnastics-style mat, a See 'n Say, LEGOs, and a crate of other assorted toys. Nearby, older children undergoing their own transfusions to combat various diseases watched videos on individual televisions.

Stacy's preparation for Katie's transfusion had begun days before. Stacy had to line up family members to take care of Calvin. She packed up food and snacks to last for hours. She mentally prepared herself to be Katie's cheerleader, to appear upbeat and unconcerned, so that Katie would think the transfusion day was a day like any other, part of her normal routine. Stacy steeled herself against her fleeting fears of blood contamination or of Katie having a reaction to the donated blood, which sometimes happened to children who had had multiple transfusions. Although the nation's blood supply was screened for viruses such as HIV and hepatitis, Stacy nevertheless felt more secure knowing that Katie got her blood from "directed donors," who had committed to donating specifically for her.

To Stacy, the day of the transfusion always seemed weighty, a reminder of Katie's struggle. The sight of someone else's blood flowing into her child's body sometimes made Stacy queasy, but she had to ignore the nausea.

Sometimes Katie tried to pull out the tubing connected to her arm. "No, no, don't pull on that," Stacy would say. Or Katie would get a toddler's impulsive idea and immediately act—like wanting another piece of chocolate and stretching toward the file cabinet, pulling her IV line taut as she sprang away from the pole. "It's a special day, girlfriend," Stacy said to Katie as her daughter went for the candy. "Don't get used to it."

"Watch, she's on the line," nurse Lori Seda warned as Katie walked toward the cabinet, nearly getting tangled in her IV line. Seda turned Katie around to free her.

Seda had become quite fond of Katie. "I didn't hear any pucker," Seda said to Katie, offering her cheek. "No chocolate then. Where's my kiss?" Katie put her own cheek out instead.

"Oh, I have to give *you* one," Seda said. She gave Katie a peck on the cheek. "Say *Lori.* You said it before. *Lori. Lori.* I heard you say it."

"Worwee," Katie said, in almost a whisper.

"There you go!" Seda said.

On each drive to the hospital, Stacy and Katie passed a playground. Every time Stacy saw all the children playing on the swings, she had the same thought: *That's where we should be, instead of heading to the hospital.* Most days Stacy refused to pity Katie or herself; she felt guilty when she did. Each visit to the hospital introduced Stacy to a new family struggling to save their child from a life-threatening disease. Stacy wouldn't allow herself to think of Katie in that category, even though in reality, Katie was.

In between transfusions, Katie seemed like a healthy child. One sunny June evening after Katie's transfusion she was playing in the backyard with Calvin and the Trebings' lumbering Saint Bernard, Hobbes (a play on the *Calvin and Hobbes* comic strip). As usual, Katie's hair was in two pigtails, with stray strands falling out the back. She was in a pink dress with frilly ruffles, barefoot, and wearing a diaper.

Katie climbed up the stairs of the yellow plastic slide and rode down. Then she ran to do it again. Until the week before a transfusion, Katie was energetic and normal. In fact, Stacy considered Katie above and beyond her age in development; she walked earlier than Calvin did, for instance. Closer to a transfusion Katie got tired, and usually got sick, a stomach virus or a fever or a cold. When Katie got weary, she had no qualms about lying down wherever she was, whether in the middle of the lawn or on a hard wooden floor.

Steve tossed a plastic baseball to Calvin, who tried to hit it with a plastic bat. "Mom, can I go to the store today?" Calvin asked. That morning, he'd found twenty dollars left by the tooth fairy—a lot more than usual because his tooth had had an infection in the root and had to be pulled. Calvin craved any attention he could get since his parents' focus was so frequently on Katie. Steve and Stacy knew that although the attention to Katie was necessary, it wasn't fair to Calvin. Steve tried to spend as much time as he could with Calvin, planning special father-son adventures such as hikes in the woods, miniature golf, and go-cart riding. Some days they'd go next door to Grandma and Grandpa's to go swimming in their pool.

Steve's friends sometimes teased him about his domestic arrangement—"You're living next to your in-laws?" But Steve loved it. Stacy's parents frequently made dinner for the young family and helped out with the kids. It had turned out to be a blessing to have family so close by to babysit Calvin when Stacy took Katie to the hospital.

Like Stacy, Steve grew up on Long Island, on its South Shore. His dad, Rich Trebing, worked for the telephone company; his mom, Kathy, focused on Steve and his sister, Nancy. Seven years earlier, his parents had bought a house on Fire Island, a sliver of a barrier beach island off the South Shore. Its streets were concrete walks and boardwalks; there were no cars; and the island was reachable primarily by ferry. Now Steve's dad was retired, and Steve's parents spent half their time at the beach house. His dad fished, his mom walked the beach. This side of the family pitched in too as the next few years unfolded.

Steve and Stacy had always wanted to have three children. But after Katie was diagnosed, they assumed they would have to put that dream on hold because Katie would need so much medical attention. But with the suggestion of preimplantation genetic diagnosis, Steve and Stacy could have that third child they'd always wanted. And, if everything came together perfectly, if one piece of the puzzle fit into another, that baby would cure their daughter. It felt to Steve like a gift. Having another child that matched Katie would set their daughter up for a bone marrow transplant should they decide to do it, like an insurance policy.

Steve stood in the kitchen later that June evening, watching Katie play with Hobbes in the yard. He cupped his hands on either side of his eyes as though wearing blinders, focusing solely on Katie. "We're doing it for her," he said. Steve resented the fact that Katie's life expectancy might be only forty years. It was unacceptable. He knew that he had to do everything possible to keep his daughter, who was joyfully frolicking in the green grass, this happy.

Steve and Stacy worried most about whether removing a cell from an embryo would be harmful to the child that grew from it, causing unforeseen health problems in the future. The Trebings learned there was no way to definitively answer that question. Pre-implantation genetic diagnosis was only a little more than fourteen years old, so the oldest people born from the process were still younger than eighteen. On top of that, there was no official database they could consult to address their concerns.

Despite the ethical issues and the unknowns, in the spring of 2004, the Trebings began their quest for the match. Regardless of how surreal the whole plan seemed, the Trebings decided they would, indeed, like to be a family of five. At the core of it all was their daughter. This plan might give her a normal life. "Although I'm not a very religious person," Stacy said, "I thought, *Should I be doing this? It's new. It's controversial. There are people who think it's not the right thing to do.* Then I look at Katie."

For Stacy, looking at her daughter made every questioning thought, all the intense worry about the right course, simply disappear. "Going through this I realized you cannot judge people unless you walk in their shoes. Never in a million years would I have thought that I would have IVF and pick an embryo out as a match for my daughter."

The Trebings would create a life to save a life.

4

"This Is a Beautiful Embryo"

At five thirty in the morning on June 21, 2004, embryologist Wayne Caswell woke up in his house on Long Island. His wife and two young sons were still sleeping. Caswell put his Chesapeake Bay retriever, Koko, in the backyard and threw the load of clothes his wife had washed the night before into the dryer. Caswell skipped breakfast, put on a black motorcycle jacket, and at six fifteen was throttling west down the Long Island Expressway on his Kawasaki.

At the office of Reproductive Specialists of New York, nine embryos waited for Caswell in two petri dishes, each dish a little smaller than the top of a soda can. These nine embryos would be tested to see which, if any, could produce a savior sibling who could change Katie Trebing's fate. When Caswell arrived at the fertility doctors' thriving office, he passed through the waiting room already filled with women struggling to have children. The embryology laboratory manager traded his leather jacket for sky blue scrubs and a blue cap to cover his hair. The hands that this morning had tossed laundry into the dryer prepared to operate on embryos so small they couldn't be seen with the unaided human eye.

Appropriately, Caswell's lab was stenciled with a playful ceiling border of sperm chasing after eggs. The nine Trebing embryos waited in an incubator that resembled a hotel room's mini refrigerator. In the petri dishes, each embryo was numbered and in its own separate drop of liquid, a drop bigger than a raindrop but smaller than a contact lens. This was the third day of the embryos' development, a critical day for the embryos, which had now grown to between six and eight cells each.

Today, the rate of cell division would increase, and the embryo's metabolic needs would change. In the body, the embryo would now normally be in the lower part of the fallopian tube, getting close to entering the uterus. So the lab was trying to do as much as possible to mimic the conditions of the female body, to trick the embryos into thinking that's exactly where they were. "We don't want the embryos to know they're outside the body," Caswell said. "We want them to think everything is normal, everything is great."

The embryos needed to be protected at all costs. The equipment in the lab was under twenty-four-hour surveillance. If the environment unexpectedly changed—the temperature in the room went up or down, for instance—Caswell would receive a message on his cell phone so he could make sure nothing was wrong. At any one time, four hundred to six hundred embryos were growing in the laboratory, awaiting the medical procedures that would help turn infertile couples into parents.

It was Caswell's job this morning to pull one cell off of each Trebing embryo. These cells would then be flown to Dr. Mark Hughes, a geneticist at Genesis Genetics Institute in Detroit, while the rest of each embryo remained growing in the incubator on Long Island. Hughes would carry out the preimplantation genetic diagnosis to find out which embryos might provide Katie with that perfect match. Caswell had one shot at taking a cell off each embryo, and Hughes had one shot at diagnosing it. It was all or nothing for both men.

Caswell had to be sure that he didn't make a mistake. As he took the first petri dish out of the incubator, he gestured to a Cornell University student working as an intern in the laboratory, asking him to verify that the dish said TREBING on the bottom in blue permanent marker. As he worked, Caswell had to be absolutely certain embryo no. 1 remained no. 1, and that its liberated cell got tagged *no. 1* as well. The numbers were how Hughes would identify to Reproductive Specialists of New York the embryos that matched Katie.

After putting on latex gloves, Caswell placed the Trebing petri dish on a staging desk, which was heated to 37 degrees Celsius, or body temperature. Caswell used a tool that worked like a miniature turkey baster to pick up embryo no. 1. He transferred it to an individual petri dish, set the embryo into a drop of mineral oil, and placed the new dish under the microscope that was the most specialized machine in the laboratory: its tabletop floated on a column of air, so if someone in the lab dropped something on the floor, the microscope wouldn't rattle while Caswell worked and cause him to destroy a precious potential life. Then Caswell placed the other embryos back in the incubator.

Seen through the microscope lens, the first eight-cell embryo looked like a soccer ball. It was round, as it was supposed to be, not flat. It was wrapped, as if in plastic, in a membrane called the zona pellucida. Caswell shot a low-intensity laser as he began to burn a hole in embryo no. 1's lining. Each time the laser was shot, it produced a bit of heat, so Caswell had to be sure not to cause thermal damage to the embryo. "One heavy shot would cause damage," Caswell said. Each cell required its own number of pulses to get a breach of the membrane. "It's not like making cookies, where it's always the same recipe." After several bursts, the embryo lining looked like someone had taken a bite out of it. Only then could Caswell steal what he was after.

One cell.

Caswell needed to pry the cell off the embryo intact. Hughes would need the cell's nucleus, what Caswell called its guts. If the cell broke as Caswell was pulling it off the embryo, the nucleus would change. Caswell also needed to take care not to damage the rest of the embryo, so that it would continue to grow normally.

Caswell considered himself a regular guy. At home, he played with his kids, and sometimes he'd trip or fall. When he tried to build something, it was never level. But in the laboratory, Caswell was a pro. He couldn't afford to be clumsy there. Caswell had learned how to biopsy embryos by practicing on mouse embryos and on human embryos that had fertilized abnormally and couldn't be used to make babies. If he damaged an embryo, he took it hard, got angry at himself, wondered if he could have done something differently or better. But he had to have a short memory as well, because he always had other embryos waiting.

"The patients have put a lot of trust in us, a lot of faith in us. They don't know who I am or what my skill level is. All of us are humbled by what we do. The work is not physically demanding, but it's mentally demanding. I'm under no illusion that I'm working as hard as a carpenter. But the mental stress of making sure I got the right cell, all that is really demanding," Caswell said. "We're basically doing microsurgery."

Most of the time Caswell didn't meet the owners of the embryos. The Trebings weren't at the lab on the day of the embryo biopsies. Steve had already left for his tent warehouse. Stacy was heading to an 8:45 a.m. dentist appointment for Calvin, and then grocery shopping. The parents, Caswell knew, would come back with the new baby in nine months to thank the doctor, to visit the nurses, but not usually to see him, tucked away in the back laboratory, behind the scenes. That was okay with Caswell; his job was not to be devoted to the parents but to the potential new child. As the doctor was to the patient, Caswell was to the embryo.

Caswell was comfortable with what he was doing with the Trebings' embryos. "My personal feeling is an embryo is a potential life. There's so much more going on with creating life than what's going on in the laboratory. I'm just assisting biology. Creating life is way beyond my control."

Reproductive Specialists of New York's lab did embryo biopsies for medical reasons only. Some laboratories in the United States had already started offering PGD for nonmedical reasons—for example, because the parents specifically wanted a boy or a girl, a concept called family balancing. "I'm not going to produce embryos just because someone wants girls," Caswell said. "We don't allow people to do sex selection."

Caswell couldn't talk while working because he used his breath to blow and suck the cell off the embryo. He used two pipettes—one to steady the embryo and the other to manipulate it. With his left hand holding the first pipette to the embryo, the second pipette went in his mouth like a straw. "I really don't like putting this in my mouth," Caswell said. "But there's no piece to do this yet." Two filters on the tube "protect the embryos from my bad breath," Caswell joked.

In a laboratory filled with sophisticated equipment, Caswell used a low-tech process that was much like sipping from a juice-box straw. First he blew, to separate the cell from the others; then he sucked, to ease the cell away from the embryo. The cell removal remained more art than science. Some cells were particularly stubborn, and Caswell needed to suck and let go, blow and let go, as the obstinate cell stretched like a water balloon, becoming more oval before it broke free and returned to a circle.

After Caswell pulled the liberated cell from embryo no. 1, he placed it in a dish and wrote Stacy Trebing's initials and *embryo no. 1* on the bottom of the dish. Then he moved on to the next embryo.

Scientists knew an embryo could survive the loss of the one cell that was necessary to perform preimplantation genetic diagnosis. During routine in vitro fertilization, embryos were often frozen for future use. One or two cells might die in the thawing process, but a fully formed human being could still grow. Nature also caused some embryos to divide into two, forming identical twins.

When Caswell got to embryo no. 4, he was pleased with how it looked. "This is a beautiful embryo," he said. It was symmetrical and didn't seem to have any cell fragmentation, which showed up as little pieces of debris in between the main cells. "The chances are that because it looks like a good embryo, it would make a baby." If the Trebings were doing in vitro fertilization only—without the added step of PGD—the embryologists would be selecting which embryos to implant merely by eyeballing them under the microscope. Embryo no. 4 seemed an ideal candidate for implantation.

But being a good-looking embryo didn't always guarantee a normal child. "It could stop growing in the next few days," Caswell said. "It could be genetically abnormal." Down syndrome embryos, for instance, grew well and didn't look any different from an unaffected embryo under a microscope.

Embryo no. 6 had perished. "It's part of the natural process," Caswell said. "Every embryo is not going to make it." Even in the human body, not every embryo makes it to a full-term baby. Some embryos have things wrong with them, and in those cases the mothers miscarry. Caswell marked embryo no. 6 as *degenerate.*

Embryo no. 8 was severely abnormal—it had advanced to only two cells. Such embryos were unlikely to survive on their own. "I can't biopsy this embryo," Caswell said. "We didn't cause that. It's just inherent in the egg. That's a hard concept for the patients. Many patients think if you've retrieved this amount of eggs, I should have this number of babies available. Problems in the eggs we can't fix. We're doing things to screen. We're doing things to select. But we're not doing things to fix."

Any embryo with fewer than five cells was not biopsied. If the embryo had only four cells, the embryologist would be taking 25 percent of it, and that made it harder to peel the cell away from the others. Plus, if an embryo had only four cells on day three, it probably wasn't a strong embryo in the first place.

By 9:20 a.m. Caswell had finished with the biopsies. Of the nine embryos, Caswell was able to remove a single cell off of seven for testing.

"Seven's not a bad number," he said.

Then he had to prepare the single cells for shipment to Hughes. He used alcohol to wipe the area where he would be working— bleach is too toxic and is dangerous to the embryos. Alcohol has a faster evaporation rate. The area had to be sterile. "It's very important for this kind of case that I not contaminate what we've done," Caswell said. "If my skin cells accidentally get in there, it might look like the embryo is an HLA match because of me."

Caswell opened a zipper sandwich bag and took out sterile

tubes that looked like they could be caps for pencils. He put one cell into each, along with a liquid called a lysis buffer, which purposely broke the cell open and suspended its DNA. Then Caswell tagged each tube with its number, deep-froze them all by immersing the tubes briefly in a vat filled with liquid nitrogen, and then placed them into a container the size of two side-by-side decks of cards. The container then went into a cooler. Caswell put the cooler in a box with regular, freezer-style ice packs. The box was marked FRAGILE, GLASS, HANDLE WITH CARE. The freezing ensured that the cells didn't get bounced around in their tubes on the journey, which could cause a cell to get stuck to the tube's lid.

Before September 11, 2001, Caswell drove the embryos to the airport himself and put them on the plane. But since then, the lab was required to use a courier service that had a relationship with the airline. So a courier was scheduled to pick up the box from Caswell at noon and drive it to John F. Kennedy International Airport, in Queens, for shipment on the next routine flight to Detroit. Caswell faxed Dr. Hughes paperwork so he knew what he would be receiving.

Now it was up to Hughes, the matchmaker.

5

"For Them, the Dice Are a Bit Loaded"

Hughes and his team had been preparing for the cells' arrival for more than eight weeks. As soon as the Trebings decided they wanted to try for an HLA-match sibling, Dr. Lipton had ordered blood samples of Steve, Stacy, and Katie to be sent to a local genetics lab. The first step was for that lab to pinpoint the Diamond Blackfan anemia gene mutation in Katie. If a geneticist couldn't find the mutation in the sick child, then Hughes couldn't look for it in the potential siblings to rule out a diseased embryo. In that case, it wasn't prudent to search for an HLA match because that match could also be born with Diamond Blackfan anemia, rendering its HLA donation useless and resulting in the family now having two children with the disease. It wouldn't even be worth getting Hughes involved.

Fortunately, Katie's mutation was in a gene called RPS 19. That was lucky for Katie—at that time, doctors knew where to find the mutation in only 25 percent of DBA patients. Because doctors knew Katie's mutation, they were able to test Steve and Stacy to see if they were DBA carriers. According to initial reports, neither of them was, so their future children had little increased statistical likelihood of having DBA. That meant Katie was most likely a random, or first-generation, mutation. Doctors don't know what causes a spontaneous mutation in a gene. It can happen at conception or because the mother was exposed to a virus during pregnancy. But this was good news: it would give the Trebings more embryos to work with because no embryos would have to be eliminated due to having the DBA mutation.

Hughes had blood samples from Stacy, Steve, and Katie delivered to his laboratory so he and his fellow scientists could double-check the genetics lab's DBA analysis themselves and then examine the HLA, the antigens that needed to be identical between Katie and the new baby.

Hughes examined each family member's DNA at the site where the Diamond Blackfan anemia occurred. Hughes had become a pro at explaining this to parents who weren't biologists.

Think of your DNA as a set of the *Encyclopedia Britannica,* he'd tell them. Each chromosome is a volume. We have forty-six chromosomes, twenty-three from mom and twenty-three from dad. In each chromosome-volume, there are genes, each of which is a paragraph long. Each has a beginning and an end. One paragraph can be one sentence long or hundreds of sentences long. For instance, the gene that mutates to cause muscular dystrophy is a paragraph that's sixteen pages long, while some genes that form parts of the hand are made up of just a few tiny phrases. The words in the paragraphs are made up of a combination of four DNA alphabet letters, A, T, G and C, which stand for the nucleotides adenine, thymine, guanine, and cytosine. The way the words are strung together tells the body how to develop.

If the mom is a carrier of an inherited disease and passes the gene for it to her child, that doesn't always mean the child gets the disease. The embryo has another correct copy of the paragraph from dad, and it can look to that copy to read the paragraph correctly. "If we are carriers, we blissfully go through life and never have any idea we have this mutation," Hughes explained. "If we reproduce with a partner who has the same mutation, then there's a problem." In that case, there's a one in four chance that a couple's baby will inherit the flawed DNA from both dad and mom. That's what happens in diseases such as cystic fibrosis and sickle cell anemia. When the DNA from mom and the DNA from dad both have a typo in the same gene paragraph, the baby doesn't have a backup copy of the gene and therefore has the disease. "Most diseases are nothing more than a typo in a single word in a single sentence in a paragraph of this huge encyclopedia of human life," Hughes explained.

Diamond Blackfan anemia is a little bit different. Even if a child has only one gene carrying the mutation, that child can still be affected by the disease—but the severity of the disease varies widely. A person who has one gene with the DBA mutation might never show any signs or symptoms, or that person might have full-blown DBA. Either way, he or she has a fifty-fifty chance of passing the defective gene to his or her child, and the child who receives it may be affected more profoundly than the parent. Why every person who has a DBA gene doesn't develop clinically apparent DBA remains a mystery that Lipton and others who work with DBA are still struggling to understand.

After he confirmed the Trebings' DBA gene results, Hughes examined the portion of the DNA that created the human leukocyte antigens.

Hughes also had become an expert at boiling down the concept of HLA matching for the parents. He'd explain that each parent has two strands of DNA, each strand containing twenty-three chromosomes, and the parent passes one of them to each child during each pregnancy. Let's call mom's HLA possibilities A and a; let's call dad's B and b. So a couple's children have four possible combinations for their inherited HLA: AB, Ab, aB, and ab. That's why statistically each sibling has a one in four chance of inheriting the same HLA as another sibling. If Katie inherited AB, for instance, in order to be a match, the new baby would also have to have those two.

Although it's possible to find a bone marrow donor in the general population, no unrelated person can be as perfect a match for a patient as a sibling. Discovering even a close match is finding a needle in a haystack.

Once Hughes knew Katie's HLA configuration and verified where her DBA mutation was, he and his lab sent the specifications to a company that built synthetic probes—fake copies of Katie's DNA that Hughes would use to compare against the embryonic cells to see if they matched. Hughes thought of them as spell-checkers.

While Hughes had been preparing for the Trebings' particular case for weeks, the technology for doing the test at all had taken years to evolve.

PGD was born in the 1990s as a way to remove a cell from an embryo so scientists could detect certain inherited diseases before a pregnancy began. Prior to that time, the only way to know whether a fetus would be born with an inherited disease or defect was to do prenatal testing on the fetus after the pregnancy was already several weeks along.

Prenatal testing began in the 1950s with the advent of amniocentesis, in which a doctor uses a needle to extract some of the amniotic fluid surrounding the fetus and then tests it for inherited diseases. Amniotic fluid is predominantly made up of the fetus's urine, which is sterile and clear at that point in the development. The baby swallows amniotic fluid and then urinates it out over and over again so the digestive system and kidneys can practice. That amniotic fluid has genetic material in it that can indicate whether the fetus has a disease or defect. But the fetus's kidneys don't form until fourteen weeks into the pregnancy, so testing can't be done until around sixteen weeks.

In the 1960s, the development of ultrasound technology allowed doctors to use sound waves to produce an image of the developing baby.

In the 1980s, chorionic villus sampling—CVS—was developed as a way to sample the placental tissue so that testing could be done earlier in a pregnancy. When the placenta is forming, it sends little corkscrew-shaped pieces of tissue into the lining of the uterus. A doctor slides a tiny catheter the diameter of a piece of pencil lead through the vagina and the cervix and touches it to the placenta at the point where it is attached to the mother's uterus. A tiny bit of that corkscrew tissue is removed. Doctors can test this tissue for genetic defects at ten or eleven weeks into a pregnancy. However, a percentage of the placenta's cells can be abnormal even if the fetus is healthy, so there's a higher false positive rate for the CVS test than for amniocentesis.

But all of these tests could only be done on women who were already pregnant, which meant that parents of an ailing fetus then had to decide whether to abort.

A couple who already had a child with an inherited genetic disease such as muscular dystrophy or cystic fibrosis had a 25 or 50 percent chance of its happening to the next child, depending on the gene. If they wanted another child, they would be throwing the genetic dice and then hoping that an amnio or some other prenatal test would show that the dice had landed the right way. "For them, the dice are a bit loaded," Hughes said.

Once the woman got pregnant, that couple would have weeks of high anxiety before a CVS test or an amniocentesis could show whether the fetus had the disease. Then they might have to decide whether to abort. "For many, that's a pathway that they're just not willing to walk," Hughes said. So the couple had to either accept having no other children or adopt.

Frustrated doctors and parents wished they could get the diagnosis before a pregnancy began.

Genetic science began to make that wish possible. The double helix was discovered by Watson and Crick in 1953, and by the 1980s scientists were finding which genes had the mutations that caused many inherited diseases. "All of a sudden people were finding genes and making associations between mutations and hereditary disease," Hughes said.

On top of that was the development of the polymerase chain reaction, or PCR, which allowed scientists to replicate DNA into millions of copies so they could be tested in a lab. That discovery won Kary Mullis the Nobel Prize in Chemistry in 1993.

To test embryonic cells, however, doctors needed access to the embryo outside of the body, before it was implanted. That's where fertility doctors—reproductive endocrinologists—came in.

In the 1970s, fertility doctors developed in vitro fertilization, in which they removed eggs from a woman's ovaries, fertilized them in a laboratory, then implanted them in the womb. IVF was first used successfully in England in 1978 with the birth of Louise Brown, who was referred to as a test-tube baby. An egg had been removed from her mother, fertilized in the laboratory with her father's sperm, and allowed to grow for three days. Then the embryo was implanted into the mother's uterus. The first IVF baby in the United States was born in 1981, conceived at the Virginia laboratory of Drs. Howard and Georgeanna Jones. Since then, more than three million babies have been born using in vitro fertilization.

The couples who use PGD to test their embryos for disease or abnormality don't necessarily need IVF, because they aren't infertile. But by using IVF, geneticists can get to an embryo before pregnancy begins. Instead of just eyeballing the embryos to choose which to transfer to the womb on day three after their fertilization, as is done for regular IVF, scientists can first pull one cell off and make a diagnosis of an inherited disease. Doctors have gotten better at nurturing the embryos in the laboratory until day five, giving them time to do the PGD testing prior to implantation.

At first, doctors used PGD to test embryonic cells in order to avoid gender-linked diseases, because testing for gender was simpler than testing for a particular gene. To eliminate the chance that parents would pass on a disease that occurred only in boys, scientists just had to identify that an embryo had a Y chromosome and then take that embryo out of the mix. That was first done in 1990 in London at the clinic of Dr. Alan Handyside. Handyside had managed to use preimplantation genetic diagnosis to test for gender and avoid adrenoleukodystrophy, also known as Lorenzo's oil disease, a nerve disorder that progresses from paralysis to death but occurs only in males.

Handyside made these strides after years of research on mouse embryos that demonstrated that cells could be safely removed from embryos for genetic analysis. Hughes believed it was also critical that Handyside was able to grow embryos in his London laboratory for much longer than anyone else had. "In my opinion, that's why it really took off at the Hammersmith Hospital," Hughes said. Handyside's laboratory worked with Robert Winston, the clinical fertility doctor who saw the patients.

"They quickly recognized that in order to be successful, this was going to require the brilliance of three different technologies," Hughes said. The ability to grow embryos to day five in the laboratory, which Handyside could do. The ability to safely biopsy embryos without harming them, which he could also do. But to go beyond selecting for gender to prevent disease, Handyside needed a genetics laboratory with the expertise to analyze DNA for a single-gene defect, like the one that caused Katie's Diamond Blackfan anemia.

A lab like Hughes's.

Hughes was identifying diseases in kidney cells in his laboratory at Baylor College of Medicine in Houston when he heard about Handyside's work. He thought testing an embryo for a disease prior to implantation could be a really exciting application of his research. But scientists have lots of ideas that seem exciting at the moment but turn out to be flops, so Hughes didn't get carried away yet.

In September of 1990, after Handyside was successful in bringing to term the first babies born using PGD to avoid gender-linked diseases, he flew to Chicago for the first International Symposium on Preimplantation Genetics, held at the Drake Hotel.

Hughes planned to attend the same meeting. "I think we both realized we had the cutting-edge technology the other didn't have," Hughes said.

But the two had yet to meet.

6

"This Is for Desperate Couples"

Dr. Hughes stood underneath the awning of the upscale Drake Hotel, waiting for a taxi. It was pouring, and he stood back from its edges so he wouldn't get wet. Hughes and his colleague John Lesko, one of the technicians in Hughes's laboratory at Baylor College of Medicine, had just attended sessions at the preimplantation genetics conference, and now they were on their way to grab lunch.

Hughes noticed Dr. Handyside also waiting for a cab.

Under the awning, the men started to talk. And they decided to go to lunch together. At a pub in Chicago, their collaboration was born.

Lesko and Hughes agreed to fly to England to help Handyside identify embryos that were free from a specific disease that was not gender-linked. They chose to start with cystic fibrosis; the genetic marker for the disease had been discovered a year earlier. People with cystic fibrosis produce thick, sticky mucus that can clog their lungs and lead to life-threatening lung infections. They have a shortened life span.

Once their first patient had gotten pregnant with an embryo that had tested free of the disease, Hughes and Handyside were hit with the monumental implications of their discovery. "We were actually doing medical diagnostics to its limit," Hughes said. "We were studying the smallest unit of life—one cell—for the smallest unit of inheritance—one gene—for cystic fibrosis—one single nucleotide letter, overnight. When you thought about it, you realized medical diagnostics would never ever be smaller than that." Hughes and Handyside wrote a paper they planned to submit to the *New England Journal of Medicine;* it gave Handyside's name first and Hughes's last, the two senior spots on a medical paper. They waited until the baby was delivered before they submitted the article so they could confirm that a healthy baby had been born. Chloe O'Brien was born in Hammersmith hospital in 1992; their article appeared on September 24 of that year.

After the publication of the paper, life got crazy for Hughes. An article on the advancement appeared on the front page of the *New York Times.* The geneticist, who was used to working in a subdued laboratory, flew to New York to appear on the *Today* show and *Good Morning America.* "It was a little bit over the top for me," Hughes said. Handyside handled the press and medical conferences in Europe. "It was a whirlwind," he agreed of the early days after their advances were published.

From the beginning, when reporters asked about the ethics of selecting disease-free embryos, Hughes replied philosophically.

"You like to do as parents what we have always done through the ages—you want your child to have a better life than you, whether you do it before they're born or all the way through college," Hughes said. "We're not screening embryos for [any and all] disease. We are testing the embryos [specifically] for what we know the parents have. Couples will always choose getting pregnant under candlelight rather than surgical light if they have the choice. This is for desperate couples."

In 1994, a desperate couple helped Hughes make a giant leap from diagnosing a disease in an embryo to identifying an HLA match. "It came from a couple, not a science mind," Hughes said. The couple had a daughter with severe combined immunodeficiency syndrome, or SCIDs (pronounced "skids"). The inherited disease has also been called the boy-in-the-bubble syndrome because people who have it are extremely susceptible to infectious diseases and have to be protected. Hughes was testing the couple's embryonic cells, sent to him by their fertility doctor, to look for an embryo free of the affliction.

Hughes by then had moved to the National Institutes of Health, in Bethesda, Maryland. He'd been recruited to be both a researcher at the NIH and the director of Georgetown University's Institute for Molecular and Human Genetics. Federal funds paid part of his salary. The father tentatively asked Hughes, "Could you test for anything else besides this gene that causes SCIDs?"

Hughes's heart dropped because he thought the father was about to ask him about gender selection or some other trait that he wouldn't find appropriate. Hughes's interest was in avoiding serious diseases. "But they had an idea that was pretty amazing: 'Suppose you could identify the embryos not only that don't have this disease, and of those that don't, you identify any of them that are HLA bone marrow matches for our daughter who is sick.'"

At that child's delivery, its family would have not only a healthy baby but also umbilical-cord blood that could be used to offer a bone marrow transplant to the sick sibling. "You literally give it to the child and take an incurable disease—an incurable disease—and cure it, just like that." Hughes snapped his fingers. "Wow.

"The more I thought about this, though, the more I worried that maybe we were crossing a line that I had drawn in my mind about testing for serious diseases and not for traits," Hughes said. Wasn't HLA a trait of no intrinsic value to that newborn baby? Would Hughes's lab be making the raison d'être of the second child saving the life of the first, and wouldn't that be wrong? "We thought about this a lot and we had conferences about this at the NIH and elsewhere with serious bioethicists discussing the appropriateness of this."

Some parents who had children with diseases that could be cured through bone marrow transplants were already trying, without the help of science, to have children who were matches. In 1990, the Ayala family in Southern California publicly declared they were conceiving a child in the hopes it would be a match for their then sixteen-year-old daughter, Anissa, who had leukemia and needed a bone marrow transplant. The Ayalas had first scoured the nation's bone marrow donor registry to try to find a match, but the number of potential donors was lower for people of Hispanic background, and they hadn't been able to secure one.

Abe Ayala went so far as to have his vasectomy reversed so he could father another child. But the Ayalas were taking a chance, hoping the new baby would be a match for their daughter. And she was. The Ayalas' case caused a press furor, with news vans parked outside the family's home; the Ayalas were advised not to take the new baby out in public for fear someone would try to take her from them. Umbilical-cord blood wasn't yet routinely used for bone marrow transplants, so at fourteen months old, Marissa Ayala donated bone marrow from her hips to her sister, Anissa, and saved her life. The family was on the cover of *Time* magazine, and their story was featured in a 1993 made-for-TV movie called *For the Love of My Child: The Anissa Ayala Story.*

"What they did was really completely just a blessing," said Anissa Ayala, who has worked for the National Marrow Donor Program in Southern California and is now the director of development for the Orange County/Empire Inland chapter of the Leukemia and Lymphoma Society. "I really feel that I'm here for a purpose, and that's really what I'm trying to fulfill." Anissa said that she is like a second mother to Marissa. "My sister is the one who will tell you that without me, she wouldn't be here, and without her, I wouldn't be here," Anissa Ayala said.

Other parents of sick children were conceiving for the same reason; in extreme cases, they tested the fetus by amniocentesis and then aborted if there wasn't an HLA match, said Arleen Auerbach, who runs the International Fanconi Anemia Registry at Rockefeller University, in Manhattan. Then they would try again. Or they would have child after child, hoping to hit the jackpot, like the Ayalas did.

PGD would merely be a more sophisticated way of accomplishing this goal, Hughes thought. It would also help couples avoid having to make the painful choice to abort. While Hughes and his colleagues were debating whether to move conception of an HLA match from a gamble to a virtual guarantee, the father of the SCIDs child came back and found Hughes in his research lab, working at a bench. "He had smoke coming out of his ears," Hughes said. Hughes took him into his office. "He hit his fist on the table and he looked at me." Hughes demonstrated. "He said, 'Damn you, Dr. Hughes, while you've been running around the world sitting around mahogany tables debating the bioethics of all of this, our daughter is dying. Give us a break. People have children for all kinds of reasons. They have them for power and money and companionship and to hold marriages together. They used to have them to work on the farm. Most of the time they have kids by accident. What's the matter with us having a baby that we're going to love very, very much who also has the miraculous power of saving the life of our daughter? How can that be bad?' This was just another example of a family who distills complicated things to their essence and puts it into perspective. They have pruned this disease from their family tree forever and also have a baby that, when it's born, they have the cord blood and can give it to the child that's sick. I don't know what's right for the general population, but I knew what was right for them."

At about the same time Hughes was working with the SCIDs family, he was sitting on a federal advisory committee that developed guidelines for the use of preimplantation genetic diagnosis and embryo testing. He thought those guidelines, which would have allowed work such as his to be funded with public dollars, would become public policy.

But in 1994, Republicans won control of Congress and refused to approve the guidelines. As of 1995, Hughes's work could only be continued using private funding.

"I went from the golden boy to the bad boy when the Republicans took the Congress two years after Clinton became president," Hughes said. Though he was working on the DNA of an embryonic cell, not the embryo itself, which in many cases was hundreds of miles away, in a laboratory, Congress still interpreted his work as embryo research. Because Hughes's salary was paid in part with federal money, his DNA work became controversial. "There were no embryos, there were no patients, there were no living cells. I was working on DNA like everyone else, whether it came from a tumor or it came from the back of your eye or anywhere else," Hughes said. He is still frustrated by what happened next.

Dr. John Wagner, who worked with Fanconi anemia patients in Minnesota, had approached Hughes and asked if he could help couples conceive children who could be bone marrow matches for their dangerously ill siblings. Hughes had begun to work with two Fanconi anemia families, the Nash family of Colorado and the Strongin-Goldberg family in New York.

"It got more and more difficult at the NIH to do this," Hughes said. "I basically was told to stop and not have any contact with these people."

At the end of 1995, Hughes left the NIH over the issue and later moved to Michigan with his wife and two young sons. It was a rough time for Hughes. His wife, Claudia, had breast cancer. Hughes was helping her battle the disease and at the same time setting up a genetics laboratory at the Wayne State University School of Medicine, in Detroit, where he could work on embryonic cells using private funding.

In January of 1998, Hughes finally resumed working with the Strongin-Goldbergs to help them try to have an HLA match to cure their son, Henry. They tried nine times, but the mother was never able to carry a pregnancy to term. Hughes was so devoted to the Strongin-Goldbergs' quest that just days after his wife died, at age forty-two, leaving him the single father to a fourth-grader and a second-grader, Hughes did PGD on a cycle of their embryos. The Strongin-Goldbergs eventually were forced to give Henry a bone marrow transplant using a donor from the general population because Henry had gotten too sick to wait any longer. The transplant failed, and Henry died.

The Nash family had moved on to work with another doctor who was doing PGD for HLA matching, Dr. Yury Verlinsky in Chicago. They conceived a boy who was born in August of 2000. His umbilical-cord blood gave his sister, Molly, who had Fanconi anemia, the bone marrow transplant she needed. She lived. Verlinsky documented and published his work, and Adam Nash is considered to be the first successful savior sibling in the world conceived through preimplantation genetic diagnosis.

By the time Hughes worked with the Trebings' embryos, in June of 2004, he had opened his private laboratory, the Genesis Genetics Institute. A courier arrived at the laboratory in Detroit with the Trebings' embryo cells the same day that Caswell had packed them up on Long Island. Hughes and his laboratory manager, Matt Studt, started working right away. They would race the clock to finish the testing—which took nineteen hours at best—in time to tell the doctors which embryos to implant in Stacy's body on day five of their development.

They opened the box that Caswell had sealed earlier and removed the seven tubes, each containing one embryonic cell. They set them in a beige machine the size of a toaster oven that could hold ninety-six such tubes at once. All of the work would be done inside these tiny tubes from Caswell.

The scientists added the probes—the spell-checkers—marked with the equivalent of the first and last sentence of the paragraphs they needed to check for the Diamond Blackfan anemia and the human leukocyte antigens. Those probes would be looking for the DNA in chromosome 19 to make sure there was no DBA mutation; they'd look at chromosome 6 to check for matching HLA to make sure the bone marrow would be a match for Katie.

Hughes also added the enzyme that caused the DNA to replicate itself. The samples were then heated and cooled repeatedly. Each time a tube was heated, the cell's two strands of DNA separated. But DNA likes to be partnered up, so as the strands cooled they looked for matching DNA to bind with, which formed more sets of identical DNA; it was sort of like running the DNA through a Xerox machine. Picture a dance floor where two people start to dance. They separate, leave the floor, and each person comes back with another partner. Then the new couples dance, separate, each of the four finds yet another partner, and all rejoin the dance floor again.

Except in DNA replication, all the couples are identical clones. This gave Hughes enough copies of each cell's DNA to test against and ensure a clear result. As the strands were heating and separating, the probes for the DBA mutation and for the HLA match went hunting through all the copies of the DNA in the embryo cell, looking for where they could bind and attach. The probes had pieces of fluorescent material on both ends, so that scientists could track the probes to see if they partnered with the original DNA.

Then the material was put into a DNA sequencer, another machine that was about the size of a thirty-two-inch television. That DNA was fluoresced with a laser so the machine could see it and translate it into the sequence of genetic letters—ATCG—that the scientists could read from a printout. Typically, the strand for HLA matching is 180 to 350 letters long. Sometimes the scientists weren't happy with the quality of the results and ran the test again. Sometimes the results were inconclusive. But most of the time, the lab was able to determine whether embryos were healthy or matches or both.

Hughes's lab charged patients thirty-five hundred dollars for a PGD cycle. "You could not do this for thirty-five hundred dollars. It's way too complicated," Hughes said. But the lab was subsidized by a nonprofit fund named for Hughes's late wife: the Claudia Hughes Memorial Foundation.

Hughes and his fellow scientists always tried not to get too attached to the results. Still, the hallway of the laboratory had a wall of fame filled with holiday cards from parents with pictures of the healthy babies born after the PGD. HLA testing was about 10 to 15 percent of Hughes's lab's caseload; the rest was testing for single-gene defects, such as the ones that caused DBA.

Once Hughes had assessed all the Trebing embryos, he would phone and fax Reproductive Specialists of New York and give Stelling—Stacy's waiting fertility doctor—the go-ahead for implanting any matching embryos.

7

"We Have Incomplete Information"

Two days after the embryos arrived in Detroit—day five of their development—Stacy was anxious but excited. Her nephew Brandon, one of her sister Lisa's sons, was graduating from elementary school that morning, but that wasn't the reason for her emotion. At noon, she was scheduled to have her embryos implanted.

Stacy ran out with Calvin and Katie to pick up balloons for Brandon's graduation. When they got back home Calvin started to cry; he'd broken the volcano he and his dad made together. "That was my special volcano," he said.

"Why don't you go color a picture for Brandon's graduation?" Stacy suggested. Calvin would be going to Brandon's graduation with Stacy's sister while Stacy went to get her embryos implanted; Steve's parents would babysit Katie.

The juxtaposition of a normal morning and the implantation was surreal for Stacy. "I'm getting my embryos put in today. Life just keeps going on even though I have this thing to do. I joke a lot and say, 'I'm going to pick up the kids today.'" But she didn't really think of the embryos that way, even though she knew some people did.

Stacy had had a dream the night before: Of the embryos tested, one was viable. It was implanted, and she got pregnant with a girl. As with many dreams, it was mixed up. In the dream, the dental hygienist from Calvin's dentist's office was the one who was checking Stacy in at Dr. Stelling's office, and she was the one who told Stacy the baby was a girl.

Steve wouldn't be going with Stacy to Stelling's office for the implantation. It was the height of the busy season for his party-tent business, and he was overseeing the installation of tents for June weddings and graduations. He'd already scheduled a week off in July to go with the family to Camp Sunshine in Maine. The camp was for families with children who had life-threatening dis-eases, devoting one week to leukemia, for instance, and another to Diamond Blackfan anemia.

With the emotional boost of her dream, Stacy felt the day held promise. Stacy and Steve's families were rooting for them. On Fa-ther's Day the previous weekend, Steve's aunt Kathy gave Stacy a candle with an angel on it. Hoping for the best, Stacy and Steve lit it the night before. They talked about all the possible scenarios for the embryos so Stacy could make decisions without him there. How many to implant if there was more than one match? Should they put in three to better the odds of at least one taking? "I don't want to jeopardize the children's lives," Stacy said then. "Triplets, you have so many possibilities of complications for the kids. If all three took, I did that. I had that choice. I put three in." Stacy and Steve decided on two maximum.

As Stacy drove to Mineola, she knew that the embryologist had been able to send cells from only seven embryos for testing, and the odds were only one in four would be a match for Katie. That was disappointing to the Trebings, because nineteen eggs had been harvested and fourteen had fertilized into embryos immediately. Stacy and Steve were surprised to learn that in the end, they had only seven from which to choose. Stelling had explained to them that this kind of attrition was normal, and it was one reason that in IVF, doctors stimulated women's ovaries to mature more than the usual one egg in a cycle.

The preparation of Steve and Stacy's embryos had begun more than a month earlier, when Stacy initially went through in vitro fertilization to surgically remove eggs from her ovaries. Embryologists normally just add sperm to the eggs in the petri dish and let them fertilize. But because these embryos had to develop without the risk of contaminating the DNA with exposure to multiple sperm, the embryologists added a step called intracytoplasmic sperm injection, or ICSI (pronounced "icksy").

After Steve gave his sperm sample, on the same day as Stacy's eggs were withdrawn, the embryologist put the sample into a solution that slowed the rate of the sperms' movement. If they swam around too quickly, it would be impossible to capture one. Under the same microscope that Caswell used to pull one cell off each embryo, an embryologist examined the sperm to select one that looked like its three parts had formed normally—a head, a neck, and a tail. Then, using a hollow needle manipulated by a controller, the embryologist quickly swiped the needle over the tail of one sperm, startling and temporarily paralyzing it. While it was still, the embryologist positioned it and sucked it into the needle tail-first so it could then be injected headfirst into an awaiting egg.

Using a pipette to hold one of Stacy's eggs in place in a petri dish under the microscope, the embryologist pushed the needle into the egg and sucked a bit of the egg's fluid up into the needle to "wake up" the egg and let it know something was occurring. Then he shot the sperm and fluid back into the egg at the position of about three o'clock. A cartoon on the wall of the lab joked about how intensely the embryologist had to concentrate during the ICSI procedure. A cat's fur stood on end, its eyes bulged, and its ears pointed up as if it had stuck a paw in an electrical socket, and the headline above the picture declared *Embryologist after ICSI.*

But once fourteen of their nineteen eggs were fertilized, the Trebings had two complications, one due to Stacy and the other due to Hughes.

Because IVF is normally done on women who have trouble getting pregnant, the amount of drugs given to stimulate the ovaries is based on the fertility challenges. The drugs can hyperstimulate a woman's ovaries, causing swelling, abdominal pain, and, in severe cases, enough fluid buildup to put pressure on the lungs and make it hard for her to breathe. In a fertile woman such as Stacy, it's more difficult for doctors to determine exactly how much of the drugs are needed.

On the night of Stacy's egg withdrawal and fertilization, Steve had an open house for his tent business. The warehouse was decorated with tent displays, and there was food in chafing dishes. Stacy was helping to host. By the end of the evening, she was doubled over and thought she would have to go to the hospital. Stacy was clearly experiencing the swelling of the ovaries. Stacy's body had to have a chance to settle down; it wouldn't be regulated in time for the fertilized embryos to be implanted five days later. On top of that, Hughes didn't have the DBA and HLA probes working together smoothly yet. He needed more time as well.

So that day the embryos had been frozen. Stacy had to wait through another ovulation cycle until her body was back to the right moment to accept an implanted embryo.

Now.

The embryos were thawed and allowed to grow to day three before Caswell took one cell from each. About 80 to 90 percent of the embryos were expected to survive the thawing process; the Trebings started out with fourteen embryos but only nine survived. So before Caswell's work had even begun, nearly half of the embryos had been eliminated.

That's why, while Caswell thought seven was a pretty good number, Stacy and Steve were disappointed.

Like the Trebings, Dr. Stelling grew up on Long Island. He went to Cornell University, and while he was in college, he was drawn to IVF, which was new and exciting and constantly in the news. Stelling went to medical school at the State University of New York at Stony Brook, where he was one of the few students in his class—possibly the only one—who knew he wanted to be a fertility doctor. He did his residency at Stony Brook as well, and he went to Beth Israel in Boston to do a fellowship in reproductive endocrinology and infertility. Stelling saw several lectures by Hughes about PGD and was intrigued by the procedure.

Stelling had married his high-school sweetheart, and they had three children, ages ten, nine, and six. One of them was born with glaucoma and had needed sixteen operations to fix it. Stelling knew the agony of wanting to heal your child. Finding the right doctor for an infant with glaucoma wasn't easy; Stelling didn't think he could have cut through the research and bureaucracy so quickly if he hadn't been a doctor himself. When he made a call, doctors got right on the phone with him. He and his wife stayed in Boston for three years because their daughter's eye doctor was there. Once they came back to Long Island, they moved back to their hometown.

"If you asked me ten years ago if I thought it was a good idea to genetically test embryos to see if one was a bone marrow match for a current child, I would have considered it an ethical debate," Stelling said. "Because you're creating life to serve a purpose outside of just being a baby. Now that I have kids, I wouldn't debate it at all. I would do it in a second. I would do whatever I could." In fact, if he was to have a fourth child and scientists could determine what gene had caused his daughter's glaucoma, he was certain he would use PGD to test his embryos to make sure a new child didn't face the same disease, even though it's not life-threatening.

Stelling was in his late thirties, with auburn hair, blue eyes, and freckles. He had been at Reproductive Specialists of New York for five years; he did an average of fifty PGD cycles a year out of the one thousand to twelve hundred IVF cycles the practice did. In about two-thirds of those fifty he was trying to find chromosomal abnormalities; in the other third he was looking for specific genetic mutations. The Trebings were one of two couples seeking HLA matches that year; the other was already pregnant.

Just before noon, Stelling sat in his office trying to call Dr. Hughes in Detroit. Stelling's PDA rested on his desk; with his right hand he was idly playing with the cap of a pen. He'd heard nothing yet from Hughes and was getting antsy so he was trying to get through to him by phone.

"Does Dr. Hughes happen to be there? I was being transferred to him, but nobody picked it up."

Caswell popped into the office to see if the results were in. Usually, the results came at the same time every day. When they didn't, Stelling and Caswell would fret. Rarely—but it happened—things went awry and Hughes couldn't get a result. The parents had a lot of time and effort invested in the attempt to get pregnant. But so did the doctors and the embryologists. When their expectations weren't met, they worried.

Stelling's voice continued. "Are we going to be happy? She's here for her transfer today. Fair enough. If there's a problem when we look at the embryos, I will let you know. But that's what we'll do."

He hung up the phone. "The results are not back," he said to Caswell. "We'll probably do the implantation tomorrow."

Caswell went to check on how the embryos were faring in the lab. As each day passed, some continued to grow healthily and some began to weaken. After too many days, the embryos would try to attach to the petri dish, sensing it was a uterus. Eventually they would perish. Also, Stacy's uterus was expecting an embryo. If one didn't arrive, she would menstruate.

Stacy had been sitting in Stelling's waiting room, and a nurse walked her down to an office so Stelling could fill her in. As Stelling approached, Stacy began apologizing for being a few minutes late. "My in-laws were half an hour late..."

She stopped talking and looked to Stelling for any indication of what the news was on the embryos.

"We have incomplete information," he told her. Hughes had tested the embryos for Diamond Blackfan anemia in his Detroit laboratory, surprising both Stelling and the Trebings. Because the previous genetic testing had indicated that neither Steve nor Stacy was a Diamond Blackfan anemia carrier, they all expected Hughes to skip that first test for DBA. But one of a geneticist's worst fears is of telling parents that an embryo is disease free and later finding out it's not. Hughes wanted to ensure the Trebings weren't so-called gonadal carriers, who have the mutation in their eggs or sperm. So he checked the embryos to make sure they didn't have the same DBA mutation that Katie did.

None of the embryos had Diamond Blackfan anemia. Those results confirmed Katie's disease was a spontaneous mutation, a random occurrence that didn't come from either parent. This meant any future children the Trebings had wouldn't have an inherited risk of Diamond Blackfan anemia. And if they needed to do another PGD cycle after this one, Hughes felt confident that there would definitely be no need to check the embryos for DBA.

But Hughes had gotten incomplete results on the human leukocyte antigen match—the news of which embryos matched Katie. He had to rerun the test, and the results wouldn't be in until eight that evening, too late to do an implantation because Stelling's staff would already have gone home for the night. Waiting another few hours until morning wouldn't have a big impact on the outcome.

Stelling's attitude was hopeful. "It's not bad news at the moment, but it's not definitely good news at the moment either," Stelling said.

But Stacy was worried. "Will waiting another day affect the viability of the embryos?" she asked.

"Only if they start to hatch," Stelling said. This is when the embryo lining breaks open completely so the cells can multiply more rapidly. "I'd rather it hatch in you, where it's used to hatching." If the embryo hatched outside the body, doctors would worry about its forming twins.

Stacy put her right hand to her face. "Wait a second. You've brought up a whole new thing here. You could put in two embryos and one could split and it could be three?"

"Yes," he said.

Just then Caswell came in to report to Stacy how the embryos were faring.

"You've been babysitting," Stacy said.

Caswell smiled. "Two are really good," he said: no. 4, which had looked so beautiful under the microscope during its biopsy, and no. 7. "Another one has grown, but it's going to be those two that we're going to hope are the matches." As for the others, Caswell wished they were a little more advanced but assured Stacy that their growth could slow down and then speed up again.

"I've seen funny-looking embryos be babies anyway," Stelling agreed, and he left to call Hughes again.

"This is killing me. I just can't believe it's only three out of the nineteen originally." Stacy's eyes were tearing.

Caswell held up a DVD.

"Pictures of the kids?" Stacy piped up, hoping to improve her own mood. "So have they been misbehaving?" she asked as she wiped her eyes.

"You're lucky," Caswell said. "Most people don't get to see their embryos."

Stacy took a sip of water from a Styrofoam cup as Caswell showed her pictures of the cells being sucked out of her embryos. He showed her embryo no. 4. "This is a good embryo," he said.

"It's hard to accept all of this attrition," Stacy said.

"As great as the laboratory is," Caswell said, "it's not as good as you."

Caswell put in another disc that Stelling's practice had made for a conference on PGD. On the tape, in the background, the Beatles song "I Am the Walrus" played: "I am the eggman, they are the eggmen. I am the walrus..."

"Bring me back to biology," Stacy said. "The sperm fertilized the egg, and that's one cell. Then it goes to two, then four? Then eight?"

On day one, the embryo advances to two cells, Caswell explained. On day two, it doubles to four cells. By day three, it should double again to eight cells; that was the day of the embryo biopsy. "We're past the stage after the eight cells. Now the cells start to talk to each other. 'You're going to be this, and I'm going to be that.'"

Stelling returned. "Are we holding up your golf game?" Stacy joked.

"Not yet," Stelling said.

"It's going to be a beautiful day," Stacy said. Today was Stelling's wedding anniversary, and he was thinking about going to the Stephen Talkhouse in the Hamptons with his wife because a friend of Jimmy Buffett's, the lead singer for the Black Crowes, would be playing there. Stelling was a huge fan, and he was hoping Buffett, who had a house in the area, would show up to play too.

"What would be easier for you tomorrow?" he asked Stacy. "Eight thirty or twelve thirty?"

They decide on eight thirty, so the embryos would be implanted that much earlier on day six in the lab.

Stelling had relayed to Hughes that nos. 4 and 7 were the best-growing embryos. "Four is half right at least," Stelling said Hughes had told him. "He didn't comment on seven. He'll have the results tomorrow."

"It's really dwindling away," Stacy said.

"One looked really good. They're done fifty percent, and so far it looks like a match," Stelling said.

Caswell tapped on the wooden desk, the knock-wood gesture so he wouldn't jinx Stacy's chances by what he was about to say. "I know it's kind of a blow that you came in today and we're sending you home, but it's not necessarily a bad thing."

But that's exactly how it felt to Stacy. Like a very bad thing.

The next day dawned with bright sunshine, and Stelling rode to the office with the top down on his convertible. By eight o'clock, Stelling was in the office, wearing short sleeves and with a beeper attached to his belt. He had already done several medical procedures and was drinking Welch's grape soda when Caswell walked in, still in his motorcycle jacket and jeans. "Get anything yet?" he asked Stelling.

"Not yet," Stelling said.

Stacy was already at Stelling's office as well, wearing a pink bathrobe and lying in a bed in the preprocedure area. A red folder that said TREBING, STACY was next to a black clipboard near the bed.

Stelling came in to brief Stacy.

"I have no news yet," Stelling said.

"He keeps it right down to the wire," Stacy said.

"I don't know about you, but I'm tortured," Stelling said. "I'm sitting by the phone that should be ringing."

"Maybe he can't get past a certain point," Stacy suggested. "I know what he's doing is very, very complicated."

"We're dealing with one cell," Stelling said. "When he calls me, I'll let you know." Stelling again went back to his office to wait.

One of the nurses had gone to high school with Stacy. They had played soccer together and hadn't seen each other in at least five years. "You look exactly the same," Stacy said to her. Except that the nurse was pregnant and due in November.

"I always have to touch the belly," Stacy said, and she did, as if hoping the pregnancy were contagious.

Every time the door opened, Stacy looked over the curtain to see if it was Stelling. When he arrived, he broke the news: only one embryo of the seven was a match for Katie, and it wasn't one of the thriving ones.

"We're going to implant that embryo and give it a chance," Stelling said.

Caswell, now in his blue scrubs, joined Stelling at Stacy's bedside. "It hasn't really grown," he said of the matching embryo. "That's not great, but it has a chance. The fact that it hasn't grown in a couple of days doesn't bode well."

Stacy tried to pin a number on it. "Ten percent chance?"

"Yeah," Caswell said. "It may do better in the uterus than it does in the lab. It's worth a transfer. Stranger things have happened."

"So it doesn't look very promising," Stacy said, more to herself than anyone. Her eyes were tearing and she walked to the nurses' station to call Steve, who was in the Hamptons putting up a tent for a graduation party. He had earlier finished putting up the VIP tent for the players at the U.S. Open.

"There's only one match and it's not a good one, but they're putting it in anyway," she said.

"All we need is one," Steve said.

When Stacy was back in bed, Stelling sat down beside her. "Three embryos are growing well today," he said. "But they're not the match. Do you want me to freeze them?"

"No," Stacy said. "What happens to the other ones? Dr. Hughes talked about donating them to research." Stacy believed the only way scientists could continue to research options for people like her was if others donated their embryos for studies. Hughes would use donated embryos to do trial runs on the probes testing for another patient's specific disease or HLA match, because if the dry run worked on an embryo, it was likely ready for use on the single cells he would be sent.

"That can be arranged," Stelling said. "Sometimes Dr. Hughes wants them. Frequently he does."

It didn't bother Stacy to reject the embryos that didn't match Katie. She didn't see them as human lives but as collections of cells with the potential to become babies. (Later, the embryos were found to have deteriorated too much to be donated to research and had to be discarded.)

Still at her bedside, Stelling told Stacy the implantation procedure would feel like a Pap smear. Stelling would insert a catheter into her uterus, and then the embryologist would send the embryo down it. They would be using the ultrasound machine so that Stelling could see inside while he placed the catheter and the released embryo.

"It's going for a little ride. Can you put a little Elmer's glue on it so it sticks?" Stacy joked. "Maybe it needs to go home. It's much better in there."

Stelling's nurses rolled Stacy's bed into the procedure room, where the staff was now in gowns and masks and booties. "I'm going to do your ultrasound while Dr. Stelling is doing your transfer," one assistant told Stacy as she rolled the ultrasound wand over Stacy's belly. Stacy had had to drink a lot of water to make her bladder full so it was easier for Stelling to see her uterus.

Three lightbulbs were on behind Stelling so he could see better. "I'm just washing your cervix off," Stelling told Stacy as he began the procedure. Then he put the tube in. Embryologist Michael Perretti slid the embryo down the catheter like a ball down a tube. They waited thirty seconds for it to settle.

"See that whiter spot right about there?" Stelling told Stacy, directing her attention to the ultrasound screen. "That's the fluid that has the embryo."

"I think I can, I think I can," Stacy chanted.

The procedure was over in five minutes. "This isn't exactly how you envisioned getting pregnant," Stelling said.

"Should I keep my pelvis up, or doesn't it matter?" Stacy asked. "Is it normal to feel a little bit of cramping?"

"Yes, some cramping is normal," Stelling said. "And you may see some spotting."

Patting her leg, he told Stacy she'd have to return for a pregnancy blood test in nine days.

"It's up to you now, and the little guy," Caswell said.

"Or girl," Stacy answered back.

At nine o'clock in the evening a few days later, after Steve and Stacy had put Calvin and Katie to bed, Stacy laid out a hypodermic needle on the kitchen counter and retrieved an ice cube from the freezer. Steve iced her lower back below the waist to help numb the coming pain.

Stacy would now endure ten weeks of shots to her buttocks. Steve jabbed Stacy with a long, thick needle filled with hormones to help the body nourish a pregnancy. The location of the shot was critical: it had to be below the waist, midway between the iliac crest and the posterior sacroiliac joint, placed into the muscle, the doctors had told Steve and Stacy. Stacy knew the anatomical landmarks from her physical therapy career, but she couldn't see the area. It was up to Steve. The names were Greek to him, and he needed guidance. The doctor had marked the area with an X in ink the first time. Steve had thought the needle would puncture the skin easily but found that the skin was tough and resistant. Stacy felt reassured that Steve played on a dart team. Transferable skills, she joked.

But on July 2, when Stacy returned to Stelling's office for a pregnancy blood test, the Trebings learned Stacy wasn't pregnant. The weak embryo didn't take. They would have to start all over again in August.

Undeterred, the Trebings headed to Camp Sunshine, saddened by their failed first attempt but still full of optimism that they would eventually conceive a match. No matter the hurdles of getting pregnant, they were convinced they would move ahead, and they felt like pioneers for a new procedure that would give hope to other families, families they would soon meet who also had children with Diamond Blackfan anemia. They weren't expecting the reaction they got at that rural camp in Maine.

8

"I Could Never Do That"

Katie threw a piece of cheese onto the examining room floor, and Dr. Lipton laughed. He knew he shouldn't encourage Katie, but he couldn't help it. She reminded him of his own granddaughter, and he wasn't good at disciplining her either. Whenever she got out of control, he and his wife would look at their watches, and say, "Oh, we've got to go." It was the privilege of being the grandparents. You could enjoy the antics. The same when you were the doctor.

The Trebings were at Schneider Children's Hospital for Katie's periodic DBA checkup, but Lipton was initially more curious about Stacy's pregnancy attempt. He had between five and eight other couples on the nationwide DBA registry who were trying to have a donor sibling as well. None of them had gotten pregnant on the first try either, as far as he knew.

"I really thought I would," Stacy said.

"Whether you get pregnant tomorrow or next year, we'll be fine," Lipton reassured her. Until Katie weighed about ninety pounds, the donor sibling's umbilical cord would provide enough stem cells for a transplant. And the life of frozen umbilical-cord blood was conservatively ten years. Katie seemed to have plenty of time.

"What are we doing until then?" Stacy asked. "What's the game plan? We talked about steroids." Doctors used steroids to try to jump-start the production of red blood cells in DBA patients. Lipton waxed and waned as a fan of steroids because, while they limited the iron buildup, they had side effects including increased risk of infection, weight gain, and mood swings. Doctors used to start steroids on DBA children in the first year of life but had found the steroids also stunted growth, and DBA patients already tended to be smaller than the norm. Katie was among the first group of DBA children whom doctors delayed starting on steroids until after they turned one, to try to alleviate the growth problem.

Katie was doing fine at the moment on the first treatment option, transfusions, but Lipton did want to try steroids on Katie before she went to a bone marrow transplant. Patients started out on a high dose for two to four weeks, then tapered to a lower dose. If the steroids induced red blood cell production at a lower dose, doctors would slowly taper Katie off of it to see if she was in remission. If Katie didn't go into remission but the steroids did make her produce red blood cells, Lipton would keep Katie on steroids indefinitely—so long as she could tolerate the effective dose without debilitating side effects—eliminating the need for blood transfusions.

Katie was playing with a blue plastic telephone, putting the receiver to her ear, oblivious to the discussion about her. Her hair, as usual, was in two pigtails. She was adorable, as even strangers told the Trebings. She was social and outgoing, and she loved to dress up in costumes and ham it up with Calvin. It didn't matter to her if it was a fairy outfit or a Batman disguise; even oversize pink sunglasses or a huge piece of costume jewelry was good enough. She was enchanted by *The Little Mermaid;* she embraced anything to do with the beach; and she couldn't get enough of either watermelon or apple juice. One of Lipton's assistants took Katie back to the playroom to choose more toys to bring to the exam room and keep her busy while the adults continued talking; Katie readily held her hand.

If Katie responded to steroids, that wouldn't dissuade Lipton from urging a transplant if a matching baby was born, he told Stacy and Steve. "I don't know that it's going to last forever," he said of steroid effectiveness. Puberty sometimes knocks children out of remission, for instance. "The clock is ticking, and then the transplant we have to do becomes riskier."

This was where Dr. Lipton and Dr. Adrianna Vlachos, the associate head of stem cell transplantation at Schneider Children's Hospital, broke ranks. Vlachos was at this appointment with the Trebings as well; she had seen up close the suffering during the transplant procedure. "If she's really in remission, people stay in remission until they're twenty-five or thirty. Why would you put her through that?" Vlachos said bluntly. Lipton and Vlachos had agreed to disagree from the moment she had joined his research team in 1992. The "dialogue" between them, Lipton found, kept him on his toes and benefited their patients in making decisions.

"This is your choice," Lipton said. "We give you the best advice we can. The issue of transplantation is a tough one. There are patients who have died. But from matched siblings, they were all older than ten. What if she's in remission until she's eleven or twelve?" Then, when she came out of remission, if they wanted to do a bone marrow transplant, Katie would be in a higher risk group due to her age.

As if to break the tension, Katie piped in. "Bye!" she yelled, causing Lipton to smile again.

"It's how you handle risk," Lipton continued. "It's a personal thing. When you have a growing, healthy thriving mermaid, you say, 'Why should I take that chance?'"

"At some point she's going to outgrow the cord," Vlachos admitted. "By then, we'll hopefully know how to manipulate the cord blood and expand it to be enough. Things are happening in real time in her life. If she's in remission and we're talking about this five years from now, it could be totally different."

This was why Lipton loved treating DBA patients. Following patients over time, establishing an ongoing relationship with them, and getting involved in their care decisions was very rewarding. He found the formation of blood the most fascinating aspect of medicine, and with the advances in science coming so rapidly, the treatment protocol was frequently changing. He loved having one foot in the clinic and the other in the laboratory. The way he treated patients in 2004 was vastly different than the way he had treated them in 1978. He and Dr. Vlachos had established a registry that would eventually follow nearly six hundred DBA patients, helping him adjust treatments as he collected data so he could offer patients the best care possible at that moment. That's how he knew that the best chance for transplant success came before the age of ten. Lipton and Vlachos both would be taking their research information to Camp Sunshine in July to lecture to the DBA families there.

Steve picked up Katie and put her on the examining table so Lipton could check her liver, palpating it to see if it seemed enlarged from iron buildup. Katie was eating goldfish. "Can I have a goldfish? Please?" Lipton said to her. Katie stuck one in Lipton's mouth.

"Start the steroids," Vlachos said. "With the steroids, she'll get very moody. If you think she's not moody already."

"Oh, great," Stacy said. "I'll be on my hormones…" Katie would have mood swings, the hormones Stacy was taking to stimulate her ovaries caused her to have mood swings as well, and even Hobbes the dog was on steroids to treat his chronic ear infections. Everyone looked at poor Steve.

"She will eat all the time," Lipton said. "She'll want hot dogs at seven in the morning and she'll eat Cheerios at eight o'clock at night."

"How much do they normally gain?" Steve asked.

"She should increase her body weight by twenty percent," Lipton said.

"I want juice," Katie said.

"We have to give her all her vaccines before we start her on steroids," Lipton said. Once she was on steroids, she would have reduced immunity, so she needed all her protection in advance.

"She's up to speed except varicella," Stacy said. The chicken pox vaccine. "Should I get her varicella?"

"Yes," Lipton said. "See you in Maine."

Stacy and Steve looked forward to Camp Sunshine as both a family vacation and a learning experience. Even Stacy's parents had volunteered as staff members, donning the pale yellow T-shirts of Camp Sunshine staff. Pam Olsen had worked as the principal of a school for the deaf on Long Island; she would help with the kids. Cal Olsen had run the nursery for years; he'd help out on the grounds. They had to arrive earlier than the DBA families. They drove up in their motor home and parked it in the lot of the camp to join the seventy-five other volunteers for orientation. They wanted to be there to learn firsthand about what their granddaughter would be going through as she grew up.

When Stacy was packing for camp in the days before departure, a sentence on the camp information forms jumped out at her: *If anyone in the family has been exposed to chicken pox within the last ten to fourteen days, please let the Camp Sunshine doctor know immediately.*

Stacy's heart sank. Stacy and Steve had just gotten Katie her chicken pox vaccine days earlier so she'd be ready to start steroids when they got home from camp. Stacy called Camp Sunshine to find out whether having the vaccine counted as having been exposed to the virus. The medical review board there decided that Katie wouldn't be able to interact with the other children because she'd had a live vaccine. Stacy and Steve could come on the campus, but Katie couldn't. Some of the DBA children at camp were on steroids, and that meant they were immunosuppressed. If a child got the chicken pox while on steroids, it would be trouble. It could spread to the child's brain or lungs. It could even be deadly. The doctors felt there was some danger that a child who had had a vaccine recently could spread the virus.

That complicated matters. Stacy's sister Lisa volunteered to go along with the Trebings to Camp Sunshine with her son Brandon. She'd watch Katie and Brandon during the day; Steve and Stacy would bring Calvin with them to the campgrounds. Camp Sunshine arranged for all the Trebings to sleep at Point Sebago, a resort property adjacent to Camp Sunshine. It wasn't the best scenario, but the Trebings didn't want to give up the chance to learn as much as they could about their daughter's disease and her future.

Camp Sunshine was started by the owners of Point Sebago in 1984. Anna Gould and her then husband, Larry, caught a television news piece about children with terminal illnesses. Anna Gould was stunned when the reporter asked an eleven-year-old boy with cancer, "How do you cope with knowing you're going to die?" The way Gould remembered it, the child answered, "I go to bed at night and pray I'm going to wake up in the morning, and I wake up and thank God I have another day." Gould's daughter, Laurie, was ten at the time. Gould couldn't imagine having a sick child. She wanted to offer children with cancer someplace to go to camp. *We've got the land,* she thought.

The Goulds were based in Boston at the time. They talked to the head of pediatric oncology at Children's Hospital Boston. They decided to print up two brochures, one advertising a camp that was just for children with cancer, the other a camp that was a family experience. Except for one person, everyone who responded wanted the family program.

As part of the program, parents were offered a group-therapy session run by a psychologist, and Anna Gould sat in. "I felt like I had no clue what these families are going through, twenty-four/ seven, three hundred and sixty-five days a year, not really knowing what tomorrow is going to bring, or the next hour, in some cases. Some of the horrific treatments they have to put these kids through…are beyond barbaric." Gould could see how beneficial the session was to the parents, who could talk without having to explain themselves. "They felt normal because they were surrounded by what their normal was," Gould said. The families also had the comfort of knowing that if something went wrong medically in the middle of the night while they were at camp, doctors were there.

The Goulds had planned to run the camp just once. But after the first week, they wanted to continue it. In the beginning, the Goulds ran the camp at Point Sebago during the off-season and funded it themselves. But as word of Camp Sunshine grew, weeks were added to offer the same program to families of children with other diseases. Funding it themselves became impossible. The Goulds set up a charitable foundation. They needed a permanent home, and in 2001 they opened Camp Sunshine on land adjacent to Point Sebago. By 2008, the camp had a $1.2 million a year budget. "We kept adding week after week," Gould said.

The gray-shingled main building has a communal dining hall, a swimming pool with locker rooms, arts and crafts rooms for the children, a nursery for the youngest kids, a library, a computer center, a teen lounge, adult meeting rooms, executive offices, and a medical clinic.

The outer buildings have forty family suites and twenty volunteer suites. The grounds boast a lake and a waterfront marina with rowboats, paddleboats, and a swim area. The camp also has a bonfire pit, a basketball court, climbing walls, a rope course, a chapel, and a small camping area with huts so the nine-to-twelve-year-olds can have campouts.

Camp Sunshine evolved into its modern form. While the children spent the days at supervised activities such as swimming, baseball, and arts and crafts, parents attended lectures on the latest treatment and research. It was like going to college for a week to study Diamond Blackfan anemia, Steve thought. All the big names in the DBA world would be there: Dr. Lipton. Dr. Vlachos. Blanche Alter from the National Cancer Institute in Maryland. People could make fifteen-minute appointments to speak with each doctor in the evenings, to ask questions specific to their cases; people who weren't from New York didn't have the luxury of periodic in-person consultations that the Trebings had.

The six of them—Steve, Stacy, Cal, Katie, Lisa, and Brandon—drove up to Maine on a Sunday in July 2004, borrowing Stacy's other sister Leslie's van because it would fit more people. It took eight hours to make the trip up through Massachusetts and deep into New England. In Maine, the winding roads were lined with fir trees and billboards with cartoon pictures of moose or lobsters.

Because Diamond Blackfan anemia was so rare, this was the first time the Trebings would get to speak in person to other parents on the same medical and emotional roller coaster. Stacy and Steve were eager to see the older children. How did they look? They knew DBA kids could be short, in part due to taking steroids, and they were curious to see how noticeable it was. In Stacy's online DBA Yahoo group, parents described the bloated moon face that steroids gave their children, and Stacy wanted to see it in person, to know what to expect when Katie started the protocol the next month. Stacy also wanted to talk to other parents about the Desferal pump that she knew Katie might have to start using soon, to get some tricks for making the daily insertion of the needle hurt less.

Stacy also looked forward to sharing the new technology they were using to create a bone marrow match. She felt sure other parents would embrace it as a wonderful thing; the almighty cure, the panacea to make the DBA just go away.

On their first night, Stacy and Steve dropped everyone else off at Point Sebago and headed over to Camp Sunshine's main building. On the front porch were bright yellow and white Adirondack chairs. Steve and Stacy loved the front doors: there were three in descending size order, as if for Papa Bear, Mama Bear, and Baby Bear. They entered through the tallest door.

Stacy's mom had been doing reconnaissance. She'd met a woman from New Jersey whose daughter had been on Desferal since she was Katie's age. When Stacy and Steve entered the communal dining hall—passing by the door with a larger-than-life blue

Sulley from *Monsters, Inc.*—Pam Olsen motioned them over to her table. She introduced Stacy to another Pam—Pam Braue Brant from Jackson, New Jersey, whose five-year-old daughter, Alexandra, had DBA. Stacy and Steve got their trays of food and sat down.

Stacy was eager to bond with another mom who not only had a daughter with DBA but also had been to Camp Sunshine before. While Steve chatted with Stacy's parents about the drive up, Stacy commiserated with Pam Braue Brant about having to stick needles into their children. Stacy felt confident enough to share her story with her.

"We're going to cure my daughter," Stacy said.

Pam was shocked. "How?" she asked, hoping she wouldn't hear Stacy say *bone marrow transplant.*

Stacy explained how she was trying to get pregnant with a donor sibling. How the first attempt had failed, but how they were going to start the second as soon as they got back from Camp Sunshine.

"You have to really think before you do this," Pam urged Stacy, surprised by how pie-in-the-sky Stacy seemed. Pam wasn't concerned about the ethics of purposely conceiving a child to be a bone marrow donor. She was worried about the possibility that Katie could die during the transplant. "Katie should really have no other alternatives before you take a chance risking her life," she continued. "I could never do that. I would not transplant my daughter. However short her time may be, at least I know she's here with me. I don't want to lose her. It's way too dangerous. I've always looked at a bone marrow transplant as a last resort. How could you risk your child's life like that?"

Stacy didn't know what to say. "But the odds are ninety percent in her favor," Stacy argued, stunned to have to convince another DBA mom. "She's young and healthy now, and she could better tolerate the transplant than if she was really sick."

"If something happened to my kid I don't think I could live with myself," Pam countered. "Don't you think you are rushing into this?" The two left their food untouched on their plates as the discussion became more intense. "Don't you want to try other options first? Are you sure you're making an informed decision? Make sure you're not just doing this because a doctor tells you this is the way to go. It's a huge decision to make." Pam didn't back down. "Transfusions aren't that terrible. There are far worse things that our kids could have."

Suddenly Stacy felt shame. Sharp tears pierced her eyes. Pam's lack of support completely deflated Stacy. She couldn't help thinking, *Am I a bad mother that I want to do this? Do I not love my child as much as she does hers?*

The answer was not that simple, as the Trebings would learn over the next few days.

9

"Why Me? Why This?"

The Trebings saw at Camp Sunshine that the life that awaited Katie wouldn't be without pitfalls if they opted not to do the bone marrow transplant. They had wanted to meet people who had grown up with DBA; people like Jen Johnson, who went to Camp Sunshine for the first time the year that Katie was born.

Jen, like Katie, had been diagnosed shortly after birth. When Jen was a child, doctors hadn't yet developed the bone marrow transplant technique to the point where the risk was worth taking for a DBA patient. When Jen was twelve, her parents did have a second child. But Jen's brother, Austin, wasn't a bone marrow match for her anyway.

Jen was in her early twenties and pretty, with straight blond hair to her shoulders. She was petite—only four foot eleven—not unusual for people with DBA. She was married and lived in Ohio with her husband, Jim, and their Jack Russell terrier, Lulu. When Jen first told Jim about her Diamond Blackfan anemia, he didn't know what she was talking about; he'd never heard of DBA, and she seemed perfectly healthy to him. But Jen knew there would soon be a night she would have a scheduled blood transfusion and wouldn't be able to go out with Jim. She also had to get home by about midnight five nights a week to use her Desferal pump. Jim needed to understand what was going on. Even though she explained her disease to Jim, it was months before Jen let Jim see her have a transfusion; she feared he'd be overwhelmed by the big bag of blood on the IV pole.

Jen was lucky in that her nurse came to her house to give her transfusions. When she was a child, her mom or dad had to take whole days off from work to bring Jen to the hospital for transfusions. Now, every two and a half weeks when Jen arrived home from work, her nurse met her there. They sat on the couch and watched TV for the two hours plus it took for each transfusion.

Jen's parents tried steroids with Jen a number of times through her childhood, but Jen didn't tolerate them well. She'd get listless, her face would become puffy, and after a few weeks, she'd have to return to blood transfusions.

The disease had taken its toll on Jen's body. Jen had already had hip replacement on one hip and would soon have it on the other. Her hips were likely damaged by either the steroids she took when she was younger or the experimental drugs she took later to try to tame the illness. Jim became the one who went down to the basement to get the laundry because climbing the steps made Jen's legs ache. Advil helped but didn't eliminate the pain. Sometimes, Jen would unexpectedly fall. Recently she'd tumbled at the mall, and Jim had to pick her up. Jim sometimes wondered if the pain would spread to Jen's knees, her ankles.

More ominously, Jen had cirrhosis of the liver. When she was growing up, Desferal came as a powder in a vial and had to be mixed first and then put in a syringe. Jen hated having to sit in the kitchen stirring it up. When she was a teenager, she sometimes skipped the protocol that was meant to protect her liver. "You want to go out with your friends and hang out. You want to be able to go to a sleepover," she said. "Your friends could stay out till midnight." She'd have to get home early to get her eight to ten hours on the pump. Plus, sticking herself with the needle in her stomach every night hurt and formed a tough callus that made inserting the needle even more painful. When she lifted her shirt, it was visible on her belly. "Nobody wants to inflict pain on themselves," she said. Even as an adult she hated doing it, and Jim and Jen would sometimes argue over Jen's reluctance. They'd get home from a night out and Jen would first have to wait an hour for the numbing agent to work before she could insert the pump. All she wanted to do was go to sleep, but she couldn't. Jim wouldn't let her; he couldn't stand to see her not do it.

"I want to go to bed," Jen would say.

"I want to see your iron levels down," Jim would counter.

Sometimes Jen would break down with Jim, asking him, "Why me? Why this?"

"Things will change," he would tell her, holding her. "A lot of very smart scientists are working on research and will come up with something." Jim hoped for a cure; Jen had been waiting for that her entire life.

For a while they struck a deal—Jim set up the pump and the medication, and Jen numbed herself and then inserted the needle.

Jen had begun taking a new medication called Exjade; it was dissolved in water and then drunk, like Alka-Seltzer. It replaced the pump, but Jim worried that the new drug might not be as effective and therefore might be cutting years off Jen's life. Jen's iron count hadn't diminished significantly, and her doctors had told her they might increase her dosage.

"I worry about the life expectancy. . . . Is there a liver transplant in her future? Is she going to have heart problems at thirty-five and we just don't know it?" Jim said. "If we have children, is she going to be around when she's fifty, or am I going to be explaining to my kids where Mom is? It concerns me a lot. I don't talk to her about it a lot, because I don't want to make her upset."

Jen's eyes teared as she listened to her husband. "I've got to take each day as it comes," she said. "I can still go to work. There are plenty of people who can't. I just don't feel like I'm ill. Then I don't know if I'm in denial. . . . I very well may be."

Her life was not centered on the disease. "It's part of my life, but it is not my life," she said. She worked as an operations coordinator in the same company where her husband was a financial planner. They were big Ohio State University football fans. They liked the outdoors, though they couldn't do as much hiking as they had in the past because of her hip surgery. They liked going to art festivals and movies.

They had started to talk about having a family. If they went ahead, they planned to use preimplantation genetic diagnosis to test their embryos for Diamond Blackfan anemia and select the ones that didn't have it. Jen's mom, Debbie Kleiber, worried about Jen carrying a baby, whether her body could handle it. Kleiber, quite frankly, just felt blessed Jen was still alive. "I feel for them because I know they definitely want a family someday. That's a huge decision, what they're going to do. I will be a worried mother. I will be worrying a lot."

Jen planned to fly back to Camp Sunshine with Jim before they started trying to conceive, to talk to the doctors there about the best way for her to achieve a pregnancy. Jim was all for that. "Are we going to bring a child into the world with this illness? No way," Jim said. "Jen is a strong woman, and very tough, and has really taken this whole thing in stride. I don't know how well I would take it. Maybe I'd still be bitter and angry at the world. Who knows if your child is that strong?"

At night, when the children at Camp Sunshine slept, the parents gathered on the deck that ran past their rooms. They had to decompress after days filled with slide shows of livers with iron overload, statistics about new drug protocols, and meetings one-on-one about their children's cases. But the Trebings missed out on that aspect of Camp Sunshine because they had to go back to Point Sebago to meet up with Katie, Lisa, and Brandon. They decided to leave a day early because it was so hard to go back and forth. Calvin kept asking why he was the only one who went to camp, why he couldn't stay and play with his sister and cousin. Leaving Lisa with three kids all day was too much to ask, Steve and Stacy decided.

Dawn Baumgardner, head of the Diamond Blackfan Anemia Foundation, intercepted the Trebings as they were heading to their van. "I know you have to go, but I want to give you this information. It's a copy of a letter I received from a family regarding transplant," she said. Steve and Stacy hugged Baumgardner, who had three sons, two of whom were affected by DBA. The Trebings took the letter and left.

Baumgardner knew it would not be an easy letter for the Trebings to read. She knew the mother who wrote it; the woman had attended camp two years earlier with her family. Baumgardner had promised the mother she would read the letter to families at Camp Sunshine; she planned to do it at a session later that day that the Trebings were going to miss, and Baumgardner knew they were seriously considering transplant. Baumgardner had to desensitize herself to the ending and had practiced reading it herself several times so she could get through it without crying.

The Trebings had piles of information and notes from the week, and they set the letter on top of the rest of the papers. Finally, when they were nearly in New York, the kids fell asleep. Lisa was driving, Steve was in the passenger seat, and Stacy was sitting in the back. They turned the radio off and Stacy started reading the five-page letter out loud. On the top, in capital letters, was typed: THINK TWICE BEFORE HAVING A BONE MARROW TRANSPLANT.

Reading just the first paragraph sickened Stacy. *Our son, Keir Zangrando, had been transfusion-dependent with Diamond Blackfan anemia since he was five and a half weeks old,* began Wendy Zangrando of Ohio. *He died on Wednesday, November 19, 2003, of complications stemming from a bone marrow transplant that was supposed to have cured him. He was twelve years old.*

As Stacy continued reading, she started to sob.

10

"I Wish We Hadn't Done It"

Keir Zangrando created a superhero with a big *A* on his chest and named him Amphibian Man. In bright colors on spiral notebook paper, Keir drew comic books of Amphibian Man slaying enemies. In episode three, Amphibian Man destroyed a monster Keir called EMLA. In episode six, he vanquished Dr. Snake Bite. When Keir's father paged through his son's drawings after Keir's death, he saw clearly that Keir used cartoons to vent his frustration with his Diamond Blackfan anemia.

EMLA was the cream Keir used to numb his thighs or abdomen before nearly nightly injections of Desferal. Dr. Snake Bite represented the nurses and doctors who poked him at monthly blood transfusions. "He had a lot of anger about his medical condition and all the things he had to go through, a lot of fears that he would express through these cartoons," David Zangrando said. Keir hated the medicines he had to take, hated the anxiety he felt about his disease, hated not being like everyone else his age. He already felt different enough from other boys: he didn't like soccer or video games. Instead, he loved Renaissance fairs. And *Lord of the Rings.* And creating fantasy worlds from everyday objects such as paper towel rolls and paint. When he had the opportunity to have a bone marrow transplant, he begged his parents to let him.

Like the Trebings, the Zangrandos had been told a transplant gave their son a greater than 90 percent chance of a cure. Like the

Trebings, they were told a transplant from an exact-match sibling was the treatment of choice for young Diamond Blackfan patients. And like the Trebings, they were told the odds of the transplant working were better before puberty. But the Zangrandos didn't have to go through what the Trebings did to have an exact-match sibling—their daughter, Emma, was born a human leukocyte antigen match to Keir, meaning their DNA shared a common trait that allowed his body to accept her bone marrow. The potential solution was at home.

When Keir was six, the Zangrandos had decided definitively against a transplant. Even the small chance that Keir could die deterred them. But when Keir was ten, Wendy wanted to go to Camp Sunshine in Maine to learn more about DBA. Even though David had already purchased four airline tickets for a family vacation in Colorado and Utah, Wendy talked him into taking the family to Camp Sunshine instead.

Keir had a great time. The DBA kids played together, showed each other how they did their Desferal pumps, felt like they weren't so different. But Mom and Dad got scared.

One of the panels at camp was made up of DBA patients in their twenties who talked about how their bodies were breaking down. They talked about how in college they hadn't wanted to be bothered with the Desferal pump, and how they now had complications such as diabetes. It spooked Wendy and David. With those stories in their heads, the Zangrandos listened to the doctors touting transplant for younger patients.

Wendy thought she was lucky to find out all this information while her son was so young, when the odds of something going wrong during his transplant seemed remote. Wendy hated that DBA required Keir to have blood transfusions—she once insisted on a vegetarian donor because she worried about mad cow disease; she constantly worried about Keir contracting AIDS. In her darkest moments, Wendy Zangrando fretted about whether a national crisis like 9/11 would prevent blood from making it to vulnerable people such as Keir. Still, making the transplant decision was agony for Wendy. She had cried when she first found out her daughter was an exact match for Keir—because that meant she'd have to make a choice.

David was an anesthesiologist. He was nervous too about doing the transplant, but he trusted the specialists recommending it. "We didn't know what the future would bring if he didn't have it," David said. "I didn't want that to happen—that in the future we'd say, 'Why didn't we do it?'" He got overwhelmed by what-ifs. What if while they were trying to decide, Emma, Keir's exact-match sister, was killed in a car accident? Then they would face the tragedy of losing both children.

Keir's eagerness to do the transplant tipped the scales in its favor. The Zangrandos scheduled the transplant for August 2003 at Children's Hospital in Cincinnati, where doctors put Emma under general anesthesia, extracted bone marrow from her hips, and transplanted it into her brother. What she remembers of the transplant is being put to sleep and later having sore hips.

After the transplant, Keir started to make red blood cells on schedule. But soon his organs started to break down; his skin produced blisters as big as Ping-Pong balls; and he needed emergency dialysis because his kidneys shut down. David Zangrando would wake up in the middle of the night and pull out his medical texts, then page the doctor on call at 3:00 a.m. with suggestions on how to help Keir.

The Zangrandos blamed their son's downturn on a drug called busulfan, which bone marrow patients take as part of the preparation protocol for the transplant. The Zangrandos said they believed the drug caused their son to contract veno-occlusive disease of the liver, which causes clots in the liver, shutting it down. One drug had the potential to treat veno-occlusive disease—defibrotide. But it wasn't yet approved by the federal Food and Drug Administration; although clinical trials were being run in Boston, the drug wasn't available at Children's Hospital in Cincinnati. David and Wendy begged Keir's doctors to get some. The doctors said it was impossible, that their hands were tied, that they could be sentenced to jail for using a drug that hadn't been approved by the FDA. Wendy didn't care. "You wouldn't go to jail to save a child?" she railed at the doctors. "My son is dying. Go to jail. I'll do what I can for you later."

Although he seemed to recover, Keir quickly got an infection, followed by pneumonia. He soon became so sick that only medications were keeping him alive. Keir began having trouble breathing and was put in an oxygen tent in intensive care. "He said, 'Why is this happening to me?'" Wendy recalled. "I said, 'They had to put oxygen on me when you were born, and I got you.'" That comforted Keir. That was the last thing his mother said to him. Keir died on November 19, 2003.

Before the transplant, the Zangrandos had won a limousine ride in a raffle. They had planned to take Keir home from the hospital in it, swinging by his school on the way to let him wave to classmates from the window. Instead, they used it to follow the hearse in Keir's funeral procession. A picture of musical instruments that Keir had drawn in third grade was etched on his gravestone. Wendy Zangrando selected a poem from his beloved *Lord of the Rings* and had it carved on his gravestone as well.

The Zangrandos were awash in regrets. David wished he'd stayed with the original vacation plan. "I feel like if I had just stuck to my guns, we wouldn't have gone to Camp Sunshine. We wouldn't have made that decision. That's the kind of what-ifs I have." He was pulled out of a depression by a stray dog that showed up on their doorstep in a red harness; red was Keir's favorite color, and he was buried in a red sweater. Wendy likes to think Keir sent the pug to them. They couldn't find the owner; the dog, which they named Pud, got David up and out of the house for walks and snored as loudly as Keir used to.

Pictures of Keir are all over the Zangrandos' house; there are twenty-one photographs of him in the master bedroom alone. Keir's bedroom is the same as it was when he checked into the hospital; his blue crayon light is still next to the bottom bunk where he slept, his *Harry Potter and the Goblet of Fire* book still under his bed, where he kept all the books he was reading. Several times Emma has donated her birthday present money to the DBA Foundation.

Wendy coped by writing the letter that Dawn Baumgardner handed the Trebings, hoping to guide people at Camp Sunshine who were thinking about the bone marrow transplant option. "It just has to be something the parents have to come to a decision about themselves, because they have to live with the consequences if it goes wrong," David said. "I wish we hadn't done it."

Stacy's voice wavered through the silent car as she continued to read from the letter, coming to the end. "'Finally, on November nineteenth, we had them stop giving him epinephrine and dopamine, the two drugs that were helping keep him alive by keeping his blood pressure normal. We spend a lot of time second-guessing ourselves. Before all this, Keir was very healthy and hardly ever got sick, not even a cold, so we feel what happened to him was really radical.

"'I think because DBA is so rare, and there aren't many sibling donors, there just aren't enough DBA patients having bone-marrow transplants for there to be reliable statistics…If the bone marrow transplant had worked, we'd be telling everyone to do it. But this is our story.'"

Stacy was crying because she felt bad for the Zangrandos. But she was also crying because now she understood she could lose her child as well. She could lose Katie.

The Trebings had arrived at Camp Sunshine optimistic and proud, feeling like pioneers with an answer to the ravages of DBA. Stacy came home depressed and afraid, even a little ashamed that she was considering a transplant for Katie. Steve felt shaken as well. They'd left for camp close to 100 percent in favor of transplant. They came home at 50 percent.

On the one hand, there was a struggle like Jen Johnson's. On the other, the chance that Katie could die, like Keir Zangrando.

And voices like Pam Braue Brant's, urging Stacy and Steve not to do it. "This is a really hard decision for you," Lisa said in the van. "You don't want to go into it with false expectations and false confidence."

After they arrived back home, Stacy and Steve hedged their bets: they would continue to try for a third child who could be Katie's donor. They wanted a third child anyway. They could decide later whether to go through with the bone marrow transplant.

11

"The Easter Bunny Would Be Jealous"

Everything during the Trebings' August IVF/PGD cycle went according to plan until the night Stacy was supposed to have an injection to ready her eggs for retrieval. Many IVF patients didn't have fertility coverage on their medical insurance plans, and the Trebings didn't either. Sometimes women who had leftover fertility medications passed them to other women who were still trying to get pregnant, saving each recipient hundreds of dollars at a time. When Stacy opened the box at the prescribed time— about 10:00 p.m.—so Steve could dart her with it, her heart sank. The syringe was empty. Someone had accidentally given her a used box.

In a panic, Stacy reached for the phone to contact the doctor on call. She'd have to wait until the next day to get the medication for the injection, the doctor told her, because it was a specialty medication that most pharmacies didn't routinely carry. Waiting drove Steve and Stacy crazy. *What if?* took over their thoughts. What if everything they'd worked for was lost by a simple mistake? The doctor tried to reassure them that the delay wouldn't scrap the entire PGD cycle, but it would push the egg retrieval back one day later than planned, and it would also push the embryo biopsy and PGD off one day as well. That one-day delay could, however, make things riskier for Stacy. It was possible another day might cause a hormonal imbalance that would hyperstimulate Stacy's ovaries, as had happened during the first round, and make the scheduled implantation impossible. But it was the only choice.

That night was one of fear and despair for Steve and Stacy. For once, they found it hard to stay positive. They felt mentally broken. They had come so far, were so close to their goal.

They followed the doctor's orders, picked up a fresh injection the next day, injected the medicine into Stacy, and hoped for the best. On Wednesday, August 18, 2004, the Trebings went to Stelling's office for the egg retrieval. Steve was exhausted. His company had installed the tents for a twenty-five-thousand-dollar-a-plate fund-raiser for presidential candidate John Kerry at the Hamptons home of Darren Star, the producer of *Sex and the City,* that was expected to net $2.5 million for the politician. Jimmy Buffett played at a thousand-dollar-a-person pre-dinner event. Steve's company put a truss system over the swimming pool, then put up the tent. Stelling, the die-hard Buffett fan, coincidentally had been eager to go to the event, but he already had a fishing trip scheduled with his son.

Stelling told Steve and Stacy he had been able to retrieve twenty-eight eggs. "The Easter Bunny would be jealous," a nurse told the Trebings. Steve wanted to know the record for the office: it was fifty-two. Which wasn't necessarily a good thing, because then there was a diminishing-returns problem. After a certain point, the more eggs a woman's body matured at once, the weaker each egg became.

An embryologist took Steve's sperm sample and, again underneath the laboratory's most powerful microscope, sucked up individual sperm and injected a single one directly into each egg to ensure the best chance of fertilization. Of the twenty-eight eggs, twenty-three fertilized.

The day of the embryo biopsies fell on August 21, a Saturday. But Caswell was in the hospital with gastrointestinal problems. And embryologist Perretti had his son's birthday party. The embryos couldn't wait. So Stelling brought in an embryologist from

Maryland, who retrieved twenty-two cells from the twenty-three embryos—three times more than the first round—and sent them to Hughes for testing. And this time, they hadn't had to be frozen because Stacy's ovaries weren't hyperstimulated, as they'd been during the first attempt; this made Steve even more optimistic. Hughes tested for HLA matches only, not for Diamond Blackfan anemia. Of the twenty-two embryos, fifteen were developing well enough to be tested as matches for Katie.

On Sunday, August 22, the night before this round's implantation, Stacy and Steve were at Steve's parents' house on Fire Island. They would leave Calvin and Katie on Fire Island with Steve's sister, Nancy, and her two children, Nicole and Jorge, while they headed back to the mainland the next day for the implantation. This time, Steve would go with Stacy.

Fascinated by what Stacy was going through, everyone wanted to watch that evening when it was time for Steve to dart Stacy with her nightly progesterone shot. The extended family gathered in the open kitchen of the beach house: Steve's parents, Stacy and Steve's niece and nephew. Stacy faced the counter, pulled the back of her khaki shorts down just a bit, and leaned over with her elbows almost in the sink. The marked ink spot had faded away, but the place for the injection was now callused from previous shots. Steve took an ice cube and held it over the area to numb it, moving the cube slightly from side to side, trying not to allow the ice to make a melted mess. He discreetly reached for the needle and aimed. With one swift motion, he hit the mark.

"Ow, Steve, you darted me," Stacy said. "It never hurts, and that one hurt." Usually once the needle was in the muscle, it didn't hurt. It was her skin that had the painful sensation.

The next morning, August 23, she and Steve headed to Stelling's office for the implantation.

Only two embryos matched Katie.

"Out of the twenty-two, I thought there'd be a lot more," Steve said. After all, the odds were that one in four would match. But, as

he'd said before, "All we need is one." Stelling implanted embryo
no. 19, which was growing so-so, and no. 21, which looked strong.

"Blackjack," Steve said.

Amid all this activity, there was still Katie's health to worry about,
and three days later—while Stacy and Steve were waiting to see
whether Stacy was pregnant—Katie had a disconcerting setback.

In her twenty months of life, Katie had already had twenty-three
blood transfusions. Each one was only a temporary fix to counter
the Diamond Blackfan anemia—each transfusion depleted itself in
three to four weeks, the length of time transfused red cells can keep
the hemoglobin at an acceptable level. After the family's return from
Camp Sunshine, doctors had started the second treatment option
on Katie—liquid steroids taken orally—to see if it spurred her body
to generate red blood cells, which would eliminate the need for
transfusions. Katie had started out taking the steroids willingly on
August 11. The family played a pantomime game: "Daddy's taking
it, Mommy's taking it, Cal's taking it." Then Katie.

But as the doctors had warned, within days the side effects of
the steroids caused Katie to be cranky and hungry. On top of these
changes, follow-up blood tests at Stony Brook University Medical
Center two weeks later—on Wednesday, August 25—showed Katie's
hemoglobin, the substance in red blood cells that carries oxygen,
had risen only slightly, meaning the steroids weren't doing much.

The doctors had hoped for an increase in what is called the
reticulocyte count. A retic count, as it's referred to, is a way of
measuring the production of young red blood cells. Katie's count
didn't even rise a half of a percent. That news was bad enough.
But the worst setback came out of nowhere: iron was building up
very rapidly in Katie's liver. Doctors and the Trebings had known
iron would build up eventually, but they hadn't expected it to
happen yet.

Ferritin is a measure of the body's total iron content; a normal ferritin level for someone Katie's age is under 400. On
earlier monitoring tests, Katie's ferritin level had been approxi-

mately 1,000, high but not alarmingly so. When the hospital called Stacy with the follow-up results, Katie's ferritin level was 4,471. To Stacy and Steve, the number seemed astronomical. It terrified them that the transfusions that were sustaining Katie's life were beginning to harm her organs.

Lipton had been talking about starting Katie on the drug Desferal, which would be administered five nights a week through a needle inserted in Katie's thigh or abdomen. But he had been waiting to see what happened with steroids first.

Stacy immediately called Lipton, and the staff put her right through to him. She was sobbing into the phone as Calvin and Katie and Stacy's sixteen-year-old niece, Samantha Giordanella, stood in their bathing suits, waiting at the door. They had been planning to head to the beach when the phone call from the hospital came.

"Don't go crazy," Lipton told Stacy. He was skeptical that Katie's counts could really be that high. The wacky results could have been caused by a virus, he said. But the only way they could tell for sure would be to put her under general anesthesia and take a piece of her liver.

"Do I need to do a liver biopsy now?" Stacy asked, distraught. The kids waited impatiently.

"No," Lipton said. Instead, they would continue with the steroids, but he would also speed up the Desferal plan and start Katie on it now. He reviewed the Desferal protocol with Stacy. "I'm here," Lipton said to her, which made Stacy feel reassured.

On the way to the beach with the kids, Stacy called the home-health-care company to set up an appointment to get a Desferal pump.

For the next few nights, Stacy went to bed crying. She hoped that her emotional state meant that she was indeed pregnant. She continued her nightly prayer: "Dear God, please watch over my children, keep them happy and healthy. Please, Lord, watch over Katie, help us to make the right decisions for her health, and please let me be pregnant with a healthy baby."

On Monday night, August 30, a nurse came to the Trebings'

house to show them how to use the Desferal pump, which was about the size of an eyeglass case. Stacy and Steve had feared this moment. Stacy pulled up Katie's pajama bottoms to expose her upper thigh. The nurse inserted the pump's needle into Katie's thigh and she screamed. Stacy held her daughter, whose body was mushrooming from the steroids, as she screamed from the Desferal injection. Soon Katie fell asleep.

Looking for some measure of hope that the future might be different from the present, Stacy went into her bathroom after the nurse left and took a home pregnancy test.

It responded with a very faint line.

Stacy took Katie and Calvin with her to Stelling's office for her official pregnancy blood test two days later, on Wednesday morning, September 1, 2004.

"Did you cheat?" the nurse asked, wondering if Stacy had taken a home pregnancy test.

"Yes! Two nights ago. It was pretty faint."

"I really think it's going to be positive," the nurse said as she drew Stacy's blood.

By eleven thirty, Stacy couldn't take the waiting anymore. She called Stelling's office for the results.

"We did it!" the nurse said.

"Woo-hoo!" Stacy yelped.

Steve was at his tent company's office. He and Stacy were taking Calvin and Katie out to his parents' beach house on Fire Island again for an extended Labor Day weekend. They would have been gone already, but Hurricane Frances was headed to Florida. Debi Pawson, who worked for Steve and whose husband, Tom, was one of the three blood donors who gave specifically for Katie, had to drive to Florida to board up the house the Pawsons owned there. Steve understood the urgency of preparing for the storm because Stacy's parents were also in Florida, boarding up their vacation home in Edgewater. Steve had delayed the Fire Island trip one day so he could cover for Pawson.

Stacy called Steve.

"You're going to be a daddy again," she said.

"Congratulations," Steve replied, breathing a sigh of relief.

Stacy decided to bring the kids over to Steve's office.

The phone rang again before Stacy could get out the door. It was Dr. Stelling.

"Congratulations," he said.

"Thank you for getting me pregnant. That sounds really weird," Stacy said.

"Everyone says that," Stelling said. "My wife doesn't mind."

Stelling reminded Stacy that she had to return to the office on Friday—she'd have to come back for a few hours from Fire Island—to take another blood test to see whether her hormones were increasing the way they should early in a pregnancy and to see if one embryo or both had taken. Stacy chose not to think about that second test.

She called her sister Lisa to tell her the news. Stacy walked back and forth to pack things while she talked on the cordless. Lisa was laughing.

Stacy called her parents at their second home in Florida. "Fill up the house," said Stacy's father. "Have more. Add an extension."

She called Steve's parents in Fire Island, but Steve had already beaten her to it. "It's official," he'd told them.

When Stacy arrived at Steve's office, he gave her a kiss and hug, but then the kids were all over him and Stacy became second fiddle.

"I'm out of here, guys," Steve called out.

12

"Come On, Baby"

The follow-up blood test to see if her pregnancy hormones were rising appropriately was just a formality, Stacy thought. She was relieved that this round of in vitro had worked. Otherwise, she knew she would have had to take a break before trying again. The shots, the emotional roller coaster of wondering whether she'd get pregnant, it was all overwhelming. Steve, as usual, was still nervous. He was in disbelief, and he wanted the test to reconfirm the pregnancy. Stacy took the 7:45 a.m. ferry for the half-hour ride from Fire Island to Long Island, leaving Calvin and Katie with Steve at the beach house.

Dr. Stelling's Stony Brook office was a low-lying red-brick building in a medical office park filled with other such buildings, making the area look like barracks. When Stacy arrived at eight thirty and walked through the glass double doors wearing a navy blue hooded sweatshirt, shorts, and black flip-flops, six other women were already waiting. Spanning one whole wall was a fish tank filled with golden fish, striped fish, black fish, white fish, nearly thirty of them. A series of rainbow paintings done by children hung near the reception desk. One picture was an American flag made of small red and blue handprints. On the counter was a hot-water dispenser and Swiss Miss packets of hot chocolate. Another counter had three photo albums with shots of children the doctors had helped conceive, a number of them photos of twins or triplets.

Woman after woman came out the reception door with a Band-Aid in the crook of her elbow. Women were dressed in workout clothes, in jeans, in dresses and shoes for work. Their hair was worn in ponytails, straight down, in clips, cut short. Regis and Kelly played on the waiting-room TV.

Stacy walked in carrying a flat box of Dunkin' Donuts for the staff. "I figure if I'm going to get fat, everyone else is too," she said, alluding to her pregnancy.

Stacy was tired. Katie had been up much of the night. Something seemed to be wrong with the Desferal pump, and Katie kept waking up screaming as if her leg was hurting. Katie was cranky anyway because of the steroids, so Stacy couldn't tell if something was really wrong. Even being at the beach didn't lift Katie's spirits.

Stacy had come to hate steroids already. She felt she was poisoning her daughter. Calvin didn't understand why his sister was hitting and biting him. Katie had zero patience. Stacy felt like strangers saw her and thought, *You should be disciplining this kid.* Stacy knew strangers looked at Katie's chubby face as she was giving her daughter another sugar-free ice pop, and she was certain they were thinking, *You shouldn't be feeding this kid.* Stacy just didn't want to get into it with people, the whole explanation of what was going on. She tried not to care what other people thought, but it was hard.

She commiserated with her online Yahoo DBA group on the computer every night after putting the kids to bed. *Katie's face is so big I think it's going to pop,* she wrote. *She seems like she can't sit still or get comfortable. She has massive mood swings where she's happy one minute and then angry the next and then weepy. I know all of these things are to be expected, but when it's your child, it is so hard to watch her like this. This has definitely been the hardest time since Katie was diagnosed. I just want to go back to transfusions, at least she was only in pain for one second when they put the IV in, now she's uncomfortable 24/7! Any insight would be appreciated.* Other DBA parents urged her through their e-mails to hang in there, that the beginning on steroids was the worst, and it got better as the dosage was adjusted over time.

If steroids were eliminated as an option, that left only transfusions or a transplant.

Which made today's results even more important.

"Any pregnancy you have could always unfortunately..." Stacy didn't finish speaking her own sentence. She'd had a miscarriage between Cal and Katie at week twelve because the fetus had had a genetic abnormality called trisomy 16. "It happens," she said.

A nurse called Stacy in.

"I feel good," Stacy told the nurse taking her blood. "Am I glowing?"

"You are a bit. Right here," the nurse said, and pointed to Stacy's cheeks.

She rubbed alcohol on the inside of Stacy's arm.

"If there are two up there, you have to go back and put in a nanny," Stacy joked, anticipating the possibility of the blood test indicating that both embryos had attached to her uterus.

Stacy had already had so many blood tests, she didn't flinch as the nurse jabbed her.

"What number am I calling today?" the nurse asked.

"I'm going to give you the cell phone," Stacy said. "I'm on Fire Island today."

"Nice weekend to do it," the nurse said.

As Stacy headed back to Fire Island, she stopped at a local Italian store to buy chicken salad, macaroni, and potato salad to bring back to Fire Island for lunch. The man behind the store's counter knew her, knew Katie because Stacy was a regular customer. He put Stacy's flyers in the store's window every time Katie's nursery school or the hospital had a blood drive in Katie's honor. "How's our little survivor?" he asked Stacy. "She kicking it? She fighting it with two fists and a smile?" Stacy felt great that she would soon be able to tell him of her successful pregnancy attempt, and the potential of healing Katie. When Stacy got off the ferry back on Fire Island, Steve, Calvin, and Katie met her on the concrete path to the house. Katie was in a stroller, in a diaper and a pink shirt that barely covered her protruding stomach. No doubt about it, she had become rotund. Calvin and Steve were in bathing suits, no shirts.

"There's no beach," Calvin said. This was the effect of the hurricane on New York: the waves had cut away at the sand, leaving a moat that Calvin had been boogie-boarding in.

"How'd it go?" Steve asked, more concerned about their personal natural phenomenon.

"I didn't get a call yet, so I don't know," Stacy said.

"No levels?" Steve asked. He was still nervous. While Stacy was contemplating the prospect of twins, Steve, ever the more anxious one, was more worried about the prospect of miscarriage.

Stacy changed the subject. "So the kids have been good for you?" she asked.

"Great," Steve said. "Katie just had three eggs, a piece of toast, and milk. Cal had a bowl of cereal."

"I fell on my knee on the cement," Calvin announced.

Stacy and Steve sat down at the table on the house's screened-in porch to have lunch. The porch was the social center of Steve's parents' beach home. A CRUST THAT'S SHARED IS FINER FOOD THAN A BANQUET SERVED IN SOLITUDE proclaimed a sign hanging on the wall. DON'T BE CRABBY, YOU'RE AT THE BEACH warned another. Seaside knickknacks haphazardly adorned the walls: A clock surrounded by seashells. A pair of swim goggles. Flamingos in a rowboat. Katie sat on Stacy's lap while she ate, and she started eating a piece of Stacy's toast.

Steve was examining the Desferal pump, trying to figure out what had gone wrong the night before. Katie's medicines were so much a part of the Trebings' lives that they didn't think twice about bringing the pump to the lunch table. "I still think it wasn't coming out," Steve said of the medication.

"I know it went on at first, because I heard it go *zzzzzzt*," Stacy said. "That's what it does when it goes on. Maybe I hit Test instead of On?"

Desferal suddenly squirted out of the pump and onto the food.

"That's nice," Stacy said. "You got Desferal in the chicken salad."

"I wanted to see if it was clogged," Steve said sheepishly. "I didn't know it was going to come out." He added, for the record, "It's not clogged."

"Susan, the nurse practitioner, said she thinks it's just one," Stacy said, bringing up the subject of potential twins.

"Two would just push us over the edge," Steve replied.

Stacy hurried to add, "Two would be exciting. But realistically, one would be more manageable, and easier with Katie."

"Cal wants a boy," Steve reported. "A brother. He says he'll watch that baby and we can watch Katie. And he'll give that baby a ride on his shoulders, because he's going to be five when it's born."

"Cal has names picked out," Stacy told Steve. "For a girl, Rebecca. For a boy, SpongeBob or Spider-Man. I like Carly, actually. Stay with the C's and K's."

Calvin and his cousins came out to the porch with ice cream cones. "What are you, crazy?" Stacy said, scolding the kids for showing the fattening treat to Katie. But it was too late. Katie ate the rest of one cousin's chocolate chip cookie dough ice cream out of a dish. It got all over her face.

"I want more," Katie said.

"There is no more," Stacy said. "You ate it all up."

Katie put the bowl to her face to drink any melted ice cream and then licked her fingers. "Done, done," she said.

After lunch, Steve took Calvin out to the ocean.

At one fifty, Stacy once again couldn't wait any longer for her test results. She called Stelling's office and was put on hold. She wiped a coffee table with Windex antibacterial on a paper towel and waited for the results.

"Should I be worried? Tuesday at nine? Okay."

She hung up. Her hormone level was only 125; the doctors wanted to see it double from the first test's level, which had been 74. Stacy would have to go back again in two days for yet another follow-up blood test.

Stacy braced herself as she went out to the beach to break the news to Steve. She knew he would take it harder than she had. Katie was whimpering in Stacy's arms and had her head on Stacy's shoulder.

"Those numbers have got me nervous now," Steve said. "They're supposed to double." This was the nightmare he'd been worrying about, that nature would betray them once again.

"It better stay," he said. He kissed Stacy on the lips.

Then he leaned down and kissed Stacy's stomach.

"Come on, baby," he urged.

13

"Take an Additional Folic Acid, in Case It's Twins"

A little before nine thirty in the morning on Friday, September 10, 2004, Stacy pulled her minivan into the parking lot of Reproductive Specialists of New York's Stony Brook office for her appointment for her first sonogram. Stacy's follow-up blood test had shown improved hormone levels, and she was solidly pregnant. Today she was having a sonogram to see whether one or both of the two implanted embryos had attached.

It had been a crazy morning and Stacy was half an hour late. She'd actually walked out of the house with her shirt on backward. Stacy and Katie and Cal waited in the sonogram exam room for the technician. Stacy put Katie in her stroller. Ever hungry due to the steroids, Katie was eating a cheese stick. Calvin sang, "Where is my cheese stick?" So Stacy gave him one too. "More, Mommy, more, Mommy," Katie demanded.

"How about grapes? Is that good?" Stacy offered.

"Yeah," Katie said.

"Cal, give this to Katie," she said, handing him red grapes. "We'll see the little swimmer in a couple of minutes," Stacy told the kids, gesturing to her belly. "Hopefully one little swimmer," she said, more for her benefit than theirs.

Sonographer Marcelo San Roman walked into the room. "You're five weeks, two days," he said. "Our main goal is to make sure the gestational sac is in the right place. We're ruling out ectopic pregnancy. That's our main goal today." An ectopic pregnancy is when the embryo develops in the fallopian tube instead of the uterus; as it grows it eventually bursts the tube and causes severe bleeding that can kill the mother.

San Roman put gel on Stacy's belly and used the wand against her skin. On the screen, shades of gray lit up. "See that dark gray? All that is the uterus," he said. "That is the gestational sac, the pregnancy," he continued, pointing elsewhere on the screen.

"How many went in?" he asked suddenly.

"Two," Stacy answered.

"See this little black circle there?" he said, pointing to the screen. "That could be a blood vessel, or it could be a second sac. Next week we'll know for sure. It's not unusual for one to take a little sooner than the other."

As much as she'd been thinking about the possibility, Stacy was still stunned when she heard she actually could be carrying twins.

"Every step of the way, you guys drive me crazy," she teased San Roman.

"Well, at least it's a short drive," San Roman said, alluding to the fact that Stacy lived only ten minutes or so from the Stony Brook office, so her coming back the next week for another sonogram to check the progress of the second sac wouldn't be so onerous. San Roman put the odds of a second baby at 30 percent.

Calvin popped out from where he'd been hiding behind the dressing curtain. "It's spooky in here," he said.

"Did you see the little sac, Cal?" Stacy asked.

"Umm-hmm," he said.

"Girl or boy, what do you want?" Stacy asked.

"Boy," Calvin said.

"Are you ready to share toys?" San Roman asked Calvin.

"Yes," Calvin said. He looked at the sonogram screen. "That is a big circle," he said.

"There's your little brother or sister cooking away," Stacy said.

"You like Barney?" San Roman asked.

"No."

"What do you like?"

"Spider-Man," said Calvin, who was wearing a blue Spider-Man T-shirt. "And Spy Kids." San Roman drew a Spider-Man in an orange dotted line on the sonogram screen over the image of the embryo sac.

Stacy dressed and waited to have her blood drawn so the doctors could check her progesterone levels. Calvin passed the time by looking for the fish that he said were always hiding in the corner of the fish tank.

"After you get your real blood taken, can I pretend to be a blood taker?" Calvin asked Stacy. He was playing with a tourniquet, tying it around his forehead. "I have a headband," he said.

"Why don't you pretend now?" Stacy said.

"You're green," Calvin said, looking at Stacy.

Stacy laughed. "My blood is green?"

"Last night I dreamed I went on a two-wheeler," Calvin said to Janet Zimlinghaus, the nurse who came to take Stacy's blood. "I went on a two-wheeler, on a bike ride. I fell off and got a bloody nose. I never like blood. I never like taking blood."

"It doesn't hurt," Zimlinghaus said.

"It does to me," Calvin said.

"It doesn't hurt at all," Stacy said. She didn't flinch as the nurse inserted the needle.

"Ohhhh, yeah, it does," Calvin said. Stacy often thought about how much more difficult things would be if Calvin were the one who was sick instead of Katie. Compared to Katie, Calvin was a chicken.

"Maybe you could put the Band-Aid on for me?" Stacy said to Calvin. "You got it. Now one for your sister. Calvin, put one on Katie.

"Do you know a due date?" Stacy asked the nurses.

"May eleventh," said Zimlinghaus.

Three days after Mother's Day.

In two weeks, if all was still well, Stacy would move on to Dr. Brian McKenna, her regular obstetrician.

"I'll be promoted," Stacy said. "Or demoted."

"Graduated," said Susan Marfoglio, the nurse practitioner.

Calvin was tying the tourniquet around his right ankle, trying to tie a bow. "I have a broken leg," he said.

"Are you taking prenatal vitamins?" Marfoglio asked Stacy.

"Yes," Stacy said.

"Take an additional folic acid, in case it's twins," Marfoglio advised.

The next week, on Wednesday, September 15, Katie had two appointments. The first was with the pediatrician, Keith Ancona. When he saw Katie, he was immediately concerned. She looked anemic to him. He wanted to get a complete blood count, but Stacy told him they had a one o'clock appointment with Dr. Lisa Mueller, Katie's hematologist at Stony Brook University Medical Center, to see how her body was reacting to steroids. Stacy was sure they would do a blood test then, and she didn't want Katie to be stuck twice in one day.

On the way to Stony Brook, Stacy and Katie stopped at the bagel store to grab lunch. But Katie also wanted the cookies and cake she saw, so Stacy ordered as fast as she could and ate in the car to get her daughter away from the sweets.

Katie had her blood drawn soon after they arrived for their appointment at Stony Brook. Katie's lips, eyelids, and fingernails were pale. Usually, after Katie had her blood drawn, Stacy would leave and the doctor would call later with the results. This time, Stacy and Katie waited at Stony Brook for them.

Normal hemoglobin is 12.5 to 14. Mueller usually transfused Katie when hers dropped to 8. Today, Katie's hemoglobin was 5.8.

They had expected Katie's level to be higher because of the steroids, because the previous week it had appeared there might be some minimal, beginning movement in Katie's red blood cell production. Her reticulocyte count had been gone up. But when

Stacy saw nurse Pattie Losquadro and Mueller coming around the corner together, she knew the news couldn't be good. Stacy toyed with the idea of running out of the room; she really, really didn't want to hear what they were going to say.

"Okay," Mueller said. "She needs to be transfused, and we need to do it today."

An unexpected transfusion; a stopgap to give Katie red blood cells because the steroids just weren't doing enough, at least not yet. Stacy asked Mueller why it had appeared briefly that the steroids might be working; Mueller said the previous test was probably a false positive.

But the pediatric hematology schedule was too busy to fit Katie in immediately. They took her vital signs to see if she could safely wait till the next day for the transfusion.

Stacy got home after four hours at the hospital, physically and mentally drained. Katie fell asleep. When Stacy called Steve to tell him that they were going to transfuse Katie the next day, she started crying. "It changes every day," Stacy said. "We think she is responding to the steroids, and now she's not. What does that mean?"

"At least we can take her off the steroids," Steve said. He hated what they did to Katie as much as Stacy did. They transformed his daughter into someone else, someone very different. But the doctor hadn't given them permission to take Katie off yet, so they still gave them to her, reluctantly. Stacy e-mailed Dr. Lipton for his opinion about what this all meant for Katie, but he didn't answer right away, as he usually did. It was Rosh Hashanah, and Stacy was pretty sure he was out for the holiday.

The next day, Katie was transfused using blood from the general population. Because the transfusion was unexpected, Stacy didn't have time to enlist one of Katie's three directed donors. That was rare and left Stacy unsettled.

Stacy and Katie were leap-frogging doctor appointments as each of them was seen once a week, Stacy to monitor her pregnancy, and Katie to monitor her steroids. On Friday, September 17, Steve met

Stacy and Katie at Stacy's next sonogram, the one to see whether she was carrying twins. Calvin was with Steve's parents, Rich and Kathy—Nanny and Poppi—on Fire Island.

As they walked into the room, nurse Fran Tulimiero said about Katie, "She looks so big all of a sudden."

Stacy answered quickly, "She's on steroids."

"No, not that," the nurse said, as embarrassed as if she'd asked a woman who wasn't pregnant when she was due. "She just looks big." She meant grown-up.

"So what are the bets?" the nurse asked, changing the subject.

"We know we have one miracle match for her," Stacy said. "I think it will be exciting if it's two. I don't want to get too excited, because I don't want to get too disappointed if it's only one." Steve and Stacy went back and forth about whether they dreaded or welcomed the idea of twins.

Steve was holding Katie, lowering her head down to the floor and back up, and she was laughing. Steve teased Katie, saying he was going to kidnap her and take him back to work with him. He had already been at work for three hours this morning, setting up a tent to accommodate a thousand guests at the next night's annual Good Samaritan Hospital fund-raising ball. It was one of forty events the company was handling that weekend. "I'll put you on my back and put up some tents."

Katie answered: "Tents!"

"Okay, we're at six weeks and two days," said sonographer Marcelo San Roman as he strode into the examining room. "Any problems?"

"No," Stacy said.

"Last week we had a gestational sac with a yolk and another possible sac. We'll know for sure today. I will show you your brother or sister because we can see it today," San Roman said to Katie. "You can see the baby. I'll be able to measure the baby from head to toe." San Roman looked at the sonogram silently. Stacy and Steve watched his every move, every gesture, waiting for an answer.

"It's just one," San Roman said finally. "That's for sure. There it is right there." He told Stacy and Steve that it was the size of a half a grain of Uncle Ben's rice.

"And it has a little heart," Stacy said. "Look, Katie, there's your miracle baby. Say hi. That was made especially for you. With love."

"Are you ready? You want to hear this?" San Roman asked.

A noise began that sounded like an astronaut communicating from the moon. Then a thumping sound began and repeated over and over.

"That's amazing," said Stacy.

Aside from the thumping, there was silence in the room.

"Even Katie's quiet," Steve said.

"Beautiful sound, right?" San Roman said.

"That is a beautiful sound," said Stacy from where she was lying on the examining table. She wiped a tear away from her eye.

Stacy put her V-neck T-shirt and her denim overall shorts back on. When she left the examining room, San Roman handed her a strip of what looked like negatives. They were ultrasound photos. "For the fridge," he said.

Stacy laughed and showed it to Katie, who had a pacifier in her mouth. "Here it is. A half a piece of rice. There's your baby."

Then she turned to Steve. "Can you believe that, that you can hear it that early?" she said. She'd gone back to look at her *What to Expect When You're Expecting* book, because she'd forgotten which stages of development happened when. This period was the development of the spinal cord, the brain, and the heart.

"It looks good. It looks really good," said Susan Marfoglio. "It's just one."

"Which is fine," Stacy said. Then she echoed Steve's refrain: "We only need one."

"We'll see you again next week," Marfoglio said. "If everything's okay, then you'll graduate."

"That'll be fun," Stacy said.

As they left, Stacy said she was relieved it was only one baby. Steve was too. "I think it would've been exciting if it was two. But when they're born, we'd be like, 'What are we, crazy?' " Steve said, smiling.

"I'm happy we got one for Katie," Stacy said. "The fact that we got one for Katie is a miracle. We could've been doing this forever."

Steve left to go back to work, but not without a reminder from Stacy. "So, are you going to call your side of the family, and I'll call mine?" Stacy said. "They're all waiting eagerly."

14

"Things Look Really Good"

Before Stacy made any of her phone calls, she went grocery shopping. She wanted to get that done before she picked up Calvin from Steve's parents, so she was racing the clock. With Katie so hungry all the time, Stacy tried to keep the house stocked with healthy choices, such as fruit. When Stacy lifted Katie to put her in the shopping-cart seat, Katie wouldn't let Stacy near her leg where the Desferal site was. "Don't touch," she said, and flinched. It was too tender from the repeated injections.

Stacy stopped at the peaches, and Katie reached up to turn her mother's face in another direction—toward a shelf piled high with bags of potato chips.

"You need the no-salt chips, girlfriend," Stacy said.

Stacy's cell phone rang. Her best friend, Maureen, had already called to find out if Stacy and Steve were expecting twins. Stacy thought, *That's probably another "enquiring mind wants to know,"* and she didn't answer the phone. Despite her obvious ambivalence about twins and her worries about both the pregnancy and caring for two more kids, she felt a little disappointed and had to tell herself it would be better to have just one so she wouldn't have to leave twins during the transplant.

"Peach? Peach?" Katie asked. Stacy gave her one. Katie took one bite and tried to throw it. Stacy caught her in midpitch, took her out of the cart, and held her on her hip as she rifled through potato chip bags, looking for the no-salt variety. So far today, Katie had eaten low-salt turkey, Muenster cheese, low-fat Vienna Fingers, grapes, a cheese stick, and no-salt potato chips. And it wasn't even noon.

Outside the store, in the parking lot, Stacy bumped into her mother.

Before her mother could even ask, Stacy held up one finger of her left hand.

Thank you, her mother mouthed to the heavens. "One. I prayed. You've already got your hands full. Congratulations."

Katie, wanting attention, threw a handful of potato chips. Pam took her from Stacy and held her. "Stop, Katie," she said. "You're feeding the birds. You're much better today." She meant after Katie's having had a transfusion yesterday.

"Isn't she?" Stacy concurred.

"Different person," Stacy's mom said.

Steve had gone back to work. His company had those forty events the coming weekend, after all. He'd started that morning at five thirty on the grounds of Good Samaritan, supervising the installation of a huge tent that had twelve peaks. Underneath, about fifteen people were working, putting up electrical lights, draping decorative material from poles, moving among the round tables.

John Lillie, one of Steve's project managers, showed up with food from McDonald's. "Oh, beautiful," Steve said, taking a large fries and a burger. "I'm really going to enjoy this sandwich."

Steve's main interest, aside from his work and home responsibilities, was darts, and he and Lillie played on a team in the Long Island Tavern Owners Darting Association league. Once a week, they met to compete at a different neighborhood bar. For Steve it was a way to catch up with his friends and take a break from reality. Steve kept his dart set in his car. He had a shelf full of trophies in his basement; his team had won the Long Island championship twice.

One dart night at a local tavern in a strip mall, Steve's team sat around a table drinking beers and eating buffalo wings as their team competed. "Things are still okay?" teammate William Drake, whom everyone called Wick, asked Steve.

"With my daughter?" Steve asked.

"With the pending child," Wick said, making a pregnant motion over his own belly.

"Everything's okay. Still pregnant," Steve said.

"Do you know what it is?" Wick asked.

"It doesn't matter," said Leanne Doherty, who often came to the dart matches to root for her friends.

"No, it doesn't matter," Steve agreed. "I didn't find out with my other two." Doherty was relieved to hear everything was going well. Whenever Steve showed up for a darts night, she was nervous about asking him how things were going. He'd had a lot of disappointment. Steve's friends usually checked with Lillie first, figuring he'd know the latest developments because he worked with Steve every day. "We ask John secretly, 'How's it going? Are they still pregnant?'" Doherty said. "We don't say a word until we get the okay from Johnny."

By late September, Stacy had come to hate steroids; Katie had been taking them for nearly six weeks.

While Katie waited to see Dr. Lisa Mueller on September 22, *All My Children* was playing on the overhead TV. This was the same unit where Katie used to get her monthly transfusions, but today the waiting room was deserted. Once in the examining room, Stacy undressed Katie and changed her diaper to make sure she'd be wearing a dry one when she got weighed so she wouldn't measure even one ounce higher than she had to. When Stacy looked at Katie, she thought Katie didn't even look like her daughter anymore, she had gained so much weight.

At twenty-one months, Katie now weighed twenty-eight pounds, six pounds more than when she began taking steroids. Normally, she would have gained half a pound in that period. She was now in the fiftieth percentile in height for her age, and in the seventy-fifth percentile for weight.

Katie's weight was just one of the issues that had been troubling Stacy lately. In retrospect, life with transfusions seemed so simple. Once a month, they'd go to Stony Brook and get, as Stacy called it, juiced up. Done.

It was more complicated now. Katie cried every night when Steve and Stacy put the Desferal needle in. Stacy wondered, *What's happening inside Katie's body that I can't see? Is her liver being damaged? What about her other organs?* Everyone was exhausted because the steroids were making Katie so hungry she'd wake up three times a night crying for a bottle of milk.

Dr. Mueller came into the examining room. She'd been Katie's hematologist since Katie was three months old. "Hey, Katie Bug," she said. She was in a long blue skirt and a white shirt; like most of the doctors Katie saw, Dr. Mueller avoided the white coat that might scare the child.

Right away, Stacy wanted to know the plan for taking Katie off steroids.

But Mueller didn't want to wean her quite yet. The steroids still might kick in. "I know you don't have hope. But I still hope she'll respond," Mueller said. Mueller wanted to test Katie's blood levels again, so Stacy sat in a chair and set Katie on her lap. Katie cried in anticipation but stuck out her arm bravely. "Even though she's crying she sticks her arm out," Mueller said. "It's incredible, because she's a little baby."

Instead of her usual rendition of "Barbara Ann," Stacy sang "Who Let the Dogs Out?" to distract Katie from the prick. Mueller joined Stacy for one bar, leaning close to Katie, and Katie smacked Mueller in the face. "You're a chunky monkey," Mueller said affectionately to Katie. She didn't mind that Katie swatted her. She knew that while the steroids made Katie moody and aggressive, they might also help her.

Swiftly, a nurse took Katie's blood.

"Okay, done?" Katie asked hopefully.

"All done," the nurse confirmed. "Good girl. You're a good girl, Katie." She put a Band-Aid on Katie's right arm.

"I want to go bye-bye," Katie said.

"In a few minutes," Stacy said.

They headed to the examining room to wait for the results of the retic count, which would show whether the steroids were spurring Katie to make her own red blood cells.

While they waited for Mueller, a medical student arrived to take more information for Katie's records. He asked Stacy how Katie was doing. "She's still a wild beast because of the steroids," Stacy said. "She's eating me out of house and home."

"Any problem as far as the medication?" the med student asked.

"I notice she shakes a lot," Stacy said. "That's new. If we're on the playground or something, her legs start to shake. Maybe it's a muscle-fatigue thing. You gain five pounds in a month, that might do it. Muscle fatigue."

"Any times you thought she'd faint or fall over?"

"No."

The student asked Stacy what other drugs Katie was on, and Stacy rattled them off. "Bactrim. Diflucan. Pepcid. Desferal subcutaneously at night. I'd like to see if I can get an order for EMLA cream because she's screaming when I'm putting it in." EMLA was a topical anesthetic. "She's on four medications. I don't like it. I feel like we're poisoning her. It's terrible. It's like she's a totally different child. It makes me crazy."

The med student left, and Stacy and Katie returned to waiting for Dr. Mueller, who had an emergency admission she had to finish. Stacy put *Barney* on the TV in the examining room and pulled a chair up for Katie. She thought about the dream she'd had last night, that she had a baby boy.

"Mommy, peach?" Katie asked.

"I don't have a peach."

"Popcorn?"

Soon Dr. Mueller entered. "Okay, Miss Muffet, can I pick you up? Can I?" She lifted Katie into her arms.

Stacy again steered the conversation toward weaning Katie from steroids.

"If her retic is up I want to leave her," Mueller said. "I want to give her the full eight-week trial. Then we can say with complete confidence that she failed or didn't fail."

Katie ate the popcorn her mother had handed her in a baggie and got it all over the examining table.

Mueller tickled Katie's tummy. "This is a big tummy. This is a big tummy," she murmured. Katie threw her McDonald's toy across the room.

Stacy asked if she should be more strict with allowing Katie to eat.

"Strict with her? Is that possible?" Mueller asked, smiling. "I think she has a mind of her own."

She told Stacy she could use EMLA cream on Katie's leg to numb the area before injecting her with Desferal, but that it might cause a rash. She suggested Stacy inject Katie in the belly instead. That made Stacy wince. "It won't hurt? I thought it would hurt because she's so distended."

"No," Mueller assured her. She checked Katie's mouth for thrush, another possible side effect of the steroids, but Katie was all clear. "So I know you don't like my plan. But I think that we should try. It's only two more weeks of suffering."

Katie turned Stacy's face toward her with her hands and said, "Bye-bye." She was more than ready to leave. Mueller played patty-cake with Katie. "She's better, don't you think?" Mueller said regarding Katie's mood. "You only tried to hit me once," she said to Katie. As if to defy Mueller's opinion, Katie hurled her binky across the room.

Stacy had to wait for the retic count before she and Katie could go home. When she heard it—just 0.1 percent, still practically nonexistent—it was the final straw. "That's terrible," Stacy said to Mueller. "Come on. You're going to wean her."

"I'm going to have to answer to Dr. Lipton," Mueller said.

"What's this doing? Really? Really?" Stacy was uncharacteristically agitated and belligerent. "I hate this drug. It's a terrible drug."

"Let me talk to Dr. Lipton," Mueller said.

Stacy couldn't stop herself. "I don't want to be six months down the road saying we didn't really give it a shot, but…but I really don't think it's doing anything. I don't care what she looks like. It's how she feels. She's up a couple of times a night. She's miserable. It's all right that she looks like a balloon. I'm sorry, I don't mean to give you a hard time. But they're not doing anything. I don't want to make the wrong decision. But the reality is, look what it's doing to her."

Mueller stuck to her guns. She knew how fast another two weeks would fly by. She'd rather see Katie respond to steroids than see her put her life at risk during a bone marrow transplant. She didn't say what was in her mind: *When Katie's lying in the hospital having a bone marrow transplant and is potentially fighting a life-threatening infection, I want to know I did everything I could.*

That night, however, Stacy didn't give Katie her dose of steroids. She and Steve unilaterally decided to wean Katie off completely. For Steve, the decision was easier. He wasn't there with Stacy at Katie's appointments every week, hearing the doctor urge them to keep going. Steve was completely done with it.

Feeling guilty, Stacy e-mailed Dr. Lipton for his opinion. She didn't want to pit one doctor against another, but she wanted his advice. He e-mailed her back that in all likelihood, if Katie hadn't responded yet, she probably wouldn't, and that he never continued steroids longer than four weeks if a child wasn't showing the desired response. But now, with the steroid option off the table, it was back to monthly blood transfusions, and maybe moving ahead to a future bone marrow transplant from the new baby.

Two days later, Stacy had her "graduation" appointment at Reproductive Specialists of New York. If she passed, she would move on
to a regular obstetrician for the remainder of the pregnancy. The
whole family went with her. The plan was that afterward they'd
go to the Central Park Zoo in Manhattan, about an hour-and-a-
half drive, to celebrate. Then they'd go to Jekyll and Hyde, Calvin's
favorite restaurant.

In the sonogram room, Calvin tried to shoot Stacy with a rubber band. "Cal, put down the weapon," Stacy ordered. "If that hits
someone in the eye, we'd have to go to the hospital and not the
zoo." From the corner of her eye, Stacy saw Steve shoot a rubber
band at Calvin.

"Did you just hit him with that rubber band?" Stacy said to
Steve.

"Yes, because he hit me," Steve said.

"Two wrongs don't make a right, Dad," Stacy said, and rolled
her eyes.

Calvin took the sky blue padded socks off the examining-table
stirrups and put them on his hands like puppets.

"Don't touch that. Dirty, smelly feet go there," Steve said.

Marcelo San Roman was on vacation in Disney World, so sonographer Cheryl Bronzino did the test.

"You feel okay?" Bronzino asked.

"More tired than usual," Stacy said.

The heartbeat began.

"Here's your heartbeat, Steve," Stacy said. "That's the heartbeat. Cal, you hear it?"

"Congratulations," Bronzino said, and gave Stacy yet another
sonogram picture.

Katie was sucking her thumb as Stacy showed her the sonogram picture. "Is it a boy or a girl?" Stacy asked Katie. She didn't
answer, so Stacy whispered, "Girl, girl, girl."

"Baby," Katie said.

"We're going to go out to the car because they're going to wreck this place," Steve said, leading a rambunctious Katie and Calvin out the door. Stacy sat in the waiting room because she had to see one of the doctors before she could officially graduate. In retrospect, the journey so far didn't seem so bad. They had started with the fertility treatments at the end of April. Five months earlier. *Other people go through much worse to have a child,* Stacy thought.

Stacy was called in, and Dr. Kristen Cain, one of Dr. Stelling's partners, came to meet her and took her into her office. The two women sat down.

"Things look really good," she said. "You've got a nice baby. It's growing well. It's doubled in size in the past week."

"Oh, so now we have a piece of rice instead of a half a piece of rice," Stacy joked.

"It's rice at seven weeks," Cain agreed. "It's a jelly bean at eight weeks, and it's a Gummi Bear at nine weeks. That's when you see the little arm and leg nubs."

Cain gave Stacy the option of stopping her progesterone shots now and switching to a vaginal suppository.

"If the shots are better, I'll just do the shots," Stacy said.

"Who is your obstetrician?"

"Dr. McKenna," Stacy said.

"When is your appointment with him?"

"October thirteenth."

"Well, what I'm going to do is write him a little letter. You are graduating. You can take these records to Dr. McKenna. You'll be able to see the umbilical cord on the ultrasound at your next visit. There'll be a big difference. It will actually look like a baby. Send us the baby picture. Let us know what's happening."

Cain stood up and walked Stacy out the door of her office. She reached to shake Stacy's hand, but Stacy pulled Cain into a hug. Tears dripped down Stacy's face.

"How do you thank someone," Stacy asked, "for giving you a child to save your other child?"

———————

Steve was outside in the minivan with the radio on; Katie and Calvin were dancing, Calvin in the front passenger seat, Katie standing
on the middle seat, facing out the back of the open hatch, yellow
pacifier in her mouth and big dimples showing as she smiled.

Stacy caught their jubilant mood as she approached the car.

"Okay, we're officially graduated," she said. "Woo-hoo!"

"Such a weight lifted," Steve said. And he drove his family to
the zoo.

15

"So Much of Who We Are Happens at the Beginning"

"Will my hands get into this at all?" Dr. Mark Hughes asked.

Hughes's face was on a TV screen in Dr. Stelling's office in Mineola, Long Island. A makeup artist was patting his cheeks with pancake to even out his skin tone for the camera. Hughes had come to New York that morning for that night's annual Kokopelli Ball, a gathering of the American Infertility Association's most eminent reproductive endocrinologists. Kokopelli is a Native American god of fertility, usually represented as a humpbacked flute player with feathers protruding from his head. For the October 4 ball, Stelling and Hughes planned to change out of their doctors' scrubs into tuxes and then take a car service to Chelsea Piers in Manhattan. Brooke Shields would be the speaker, talking to the 550 attendees about her struggles with infertility.

But Stelling capitalized on Hughes's trip to New York by asking him to help Reproductive Specialists of New York film a DVD that explained preimplantation genetic diagnosis. The DVD would be given to patients who had chromosomal abnormalities, carried genetic defects, or, like the Trebings, needed a bone marrow match for a sick sibling, and the patients could take it home, watch it, digest it, watch it again, then ask any questions and make their decisions.

The Trebings had been asked to appear on the DVD as well. They were thrilled—that meant they would get to meet Hughes, whom they considered a genius. They were set to arrive at Stelling's office in Mineola later in the day.

"Are you going to ask me questions, or am I just going to start yapping?" Hughes asked, his shoes kicked off under the table.

"I'm going to ask you questions," said Craig Cooper of 30fps Productions/Promotion Associates. "They will not hear my questions in the video. When I ask you, 'What was reproductive endocrinology like fifteen years ago?' don't say, 'It was...' because they won't hear my questions. Start with something like 'Reproductive endocrinology...' Okay. Give me the thirty- to sixty-second synopsis of the field of PGD."

Hughes began, using his usual encyclopedia metaphor to explain how embryos were tested for disease or screened for chromosomal abnormalities or for HLA matching.

Cooper interjected. "I have picked up on twinges of controversy in talking to some folks. That there are people who have a problem with some of what it is that you're doing."

"New things are controversial. New things are scary," Hughes said. He cited the controversy over the first heart transplant when it was performed in 1967 by South African surgeon Christiaan Barnard, how people said it would be a fountain of youth available only to the rich. Now many people choose to sign the back of their driver's licenses to donate their organs.

Hughes acknowledged that some Americans thought embryos deserved the same rights as human beings and that scientists shouldn't be testing them and choosing which to implant, then discarding the excess embryos that had been created in the process.

"If you believe the fertilized egg has the same ethical value as the toddler on the swing set in the backyard, then you would say that all of this is inappropriate," Hughes said. "But then you would also have to say IVF is inappropriate. In IVF, for twenty-five years, embryos have been selected. The ones that are growing the best are transferred to the womb." In regular IVF, embryologists look at embryos under a microscope and decide which ones to implant and which to discard or freeze for possible future use by the couple. With PGD, they look at the DNA. "Now we have the ability to look at it genetically. The measuring stick has changed."

"If you can do that, might you also select traits, and traits that are of no intrinsic value to the newborn baby but are of value to a sibling who needs a bone marrow transplant? Or for gender?" Cooper asked.

Indeed, some bioethicists worried that people might start to want their embryos' DNA tested for traits such as eye color or height or musical ability, Hughes agreed. "Any technology can be abused. That's not what makes it right or wrong. How do you do it in an ethical way? It's quite complicated."

Cooper stopped to switch tapes. "This is good stuff. Very good stuff," he said. He continued to question Hughes. "How do you know that taking this cell from the embryo isn't going to do damage?" Cooper asked.

"Every couple has a background risk of having a birth defect. No one is guaranteeing perfection here. There are risks. There have been errors in PGD at every laboratory in the world that does this. The goal here is to change their odds a lot. But not zero. Zero is perfect. As soon as you begin to think that you can be perfect, Mother Nature is going to throw you a curveball."

Cooper had Hughes take a break.

"You all right?" Cooper said. "You want a drink?"

"Maybe if there's some water out here. How are we doing?"

"We're doing awesome," Cooper said.

Stelling and his colleague Dr. Gabriel San Roman were watching the filming. "Have you seen Stacy?" Stelling asked San Roman. She and Steve were supposed to arrive soon.

"No, I haven't seen her yet," San Roman said.

As if on cue, Stacy and Steve showed up. They waited outside the filming room to meet Hughes. Stacy looked pregnant now. She and Steve were both dressed fashionably, avoiding their usual jeans. Stacy was in a striped blouse; she had styled her short hair with mousse. Steve had gotten a haircut.

Stacy kissed Dr. Stelling hello. Then Dr. Hughes emerged from the filming room.

"I am so happy for you," he said to Stacy and Steve. "Good to meet you."

"Thank you," Stacy said. "Katie thanks you. Very much. I can't thank you enough. I can't thank Dr. Stelling enough. I told myself I'm not going to cry today. I'm going to try really hard. It's really a pleasure to meet you. I'm so glad there are geniuses in the world."

"Such as yourself," Steve said.

"This is what it's all about," Hughes said, beaming. "I went into medicine and science to do exactly this. To see smiles on your faces and healthy babies in your arms. That's what it's all about. So you'll have a CVS or an amnio coming up, right?"

Stacy was flustered. "Um, well, I don't know." She glanced at Steve. "We haven't really discussed whether or not…," Stacy said.

"You usually would," Stelling broke in.

"This is very complicated stuff. You want to be sure," Hughes said. "There have been errors. You don't want them to happen to you. We want to know."

"When do they normally do the tests?" Stacy asked.

"CVS is around ten to twelve weeks. Amnio is around fourteen or fifteen weeks," Stelling said.

"I don't know what a CVS is," Stacy said.

"Chorionic villus sampling. It's like an amnio, but you do it earlier by testing the placenta," Hughes said.

But Stacy knew she wouldn't do amniocentesis or CVS. She was having the child no matter what. It might not be a match, but this far along in a pregnancy, Stacy knew she wouldn't terminate because of a matching error. She wasn't willing to risk any complications an amnio might cause just to find out information she wouldn't act on anyway.

Another couple, Lynette and Jeremy Mutschler, joined them. The Mutschlers were trying to avoid with their next child an inherited disease that they had passed to their daughter, who had lived for just one day. Lynette just had her implantation a few days earlier. "Today's the first day my husband's letting me walk," she said.

"I don't want to take any chances," Jeremy said.

"Good luck," Stacy said. "Has it been a rough road?"

"About five years of a rough road," Lynette said. "It's just amazing, this technology."

"I'll put on my political hat for a minute," Hughes said. "Isn't it amazing that there are people who want to ban this? What could be more American than creating healthy families?"

"Maybe you should send this DVD to the White House," Stacy said. To President George W. Bush.

"I don't want to get anywhere near the White House," Hughes said. "I went from a golden boy to a bad boy when the political climate changed in the United States."

"It'll change again," Stacy said.

"There haven't been enough people who have walked in our shoes," Lynette said. "Anybody, anybody would do what we're doing for our children. There's not an ounce of me that could bury another child."

"All they have to do is change their circumstances, change their situations, and they would change their tunes," Steve said.

"Do you think people will select for traits?" Hughes said. "I don't care if you're a multimillionaire. Who would go through this if they didn't have to? Let's get real. Long fingers to be a pianist? It's not one gene. It's a blend of genes."

Cooper interrupted to tell them he was ready to videotape Stacy having an ultrasound so they could show the heart beating. Hughes and Stelling left to change into royal blue scrubs.

Hughes and Stelling chatted as they waited for Stacy to get ready and for Cooper to finish setting up the lighting in the ultrasound room. "My car license plate says DNA DOC," Hughes said.

"I thought about being PGD DOC or IVF DOC or PGD TIME," Stelling said.

"Most people would have no clue what PGD was," Hughes said. "IVF they would, but not PGD. Figure this one out." Hughes wrote down a possible license plate on a piece of paper: OBIGYNOB. It was a play on the Star Wars Jedi knight character Obi-Wan Kenobi. "I saw one once, it was REPRO MAN," Hughes said.

"There's a lot of them you can't stick on there. Like THE INSEMI-NATOR," Stelling said. Stelling owned a boat he'd named *Fishing for Follicles*. He meant, of course, the eggs he retrieved from fertility patients, but most fellow boaters thought the name referred to hair loss.

As the doctors were talking, a nurse in scrubs approached and handed Stelling a piece of paper. On it was the name of a patient he'd done PGD for to avoid inherited disease; the parents had just called to report mom had given birth to a healthy baby boy that day. *PGD baby boy Jake Matthew, 7 lbs., 7 oz., 21 inches long,* the message said.

Stacy was stretched out on a table in the sonogram room, the lower half of her body covered by a sheet. Cathy Dennis, a nurse practitioner and Stelling's sister, was in the room to do the sonogram. Steve, Stelling, and Hughes all watched.

The heartbeat began.

"I always like hearing that sound," Stelling said.

"That sounds great," Stacy said.

"A carpenter would say it's cutting a log," Hughes said.

"It's the sound of life to me," Stacy said.

"It is, it's wonderful," Hughes said.

"It's the product of both of you," Stacy said to Stelling and Hughes.

"No, this is your product," Hughes said. "I'm just an assistant. See the arm?"

"I can't see the arm," Stacy said.

"It's this little thing right here," Stelling said, pointing.

"It's just a miracle," Stacy said.

"The whole thing is a miracle. Whether you do it by yourself or you do it in the clinic, it's a miracle. Just a miracle," Hughes agreed.

"Can you see, hon?" Stacy said to Steve, who was standing across the room trying not to get in the way of the cameras.

"Dad, you're supposed to be over here," Hughes said. Steve came closer to the sonogram screen. Stacy lifted her arms off the table in triumph. "My three men. These are my three men," she said, laughing.

"Our part's over," Stelling said. "His part's just beginning."

After the sonogram, it was Stacy and Steve's turn to be interviewed by Cooper. Stacy explained the three treatment options for Diamond Blackfan anemia: transfusions supplemented by Desferal; steroids; or a bone marrow transplant from an exact-match sibling.

"What went through your minds when option three was a possibility?" Cooper asked.

"As parents we felt we would want to do anything we possibly could for our daughter," Steve said. "As a parent, it hurts. Anything we could possibly do to cure her, we'd strive for. Fortunately, we're blessed with having a direct match now for our daughter.

"There is controversy over what we're doing," Steve continued. "Personally, I haven't had any negative feedback. Perhaps those people are not parents and they are not faced with the situation we're in."

Stacy broke in. "I'm very open about it," she said. "I have had one situation." She explained that she was telling a woman about their IVF with PGD to conceive a donor sibling. The woman said to Stacy, "Make sure you don't say that to your child, the child you're carrying." But Stacy couldn't relate to what she was saying.

Stacy looked at it so much differently. "Every child is a miracle," Stacy said. "This child is going to be a miracle just like my other two children are. The fact that this child would be a match for my daughter is just another miracle. So we would be doubly blessed."

Steve took over again. "Dr. Hughes is a genius," he said.

Stacy agreed. "He's just one of those people who is going to make history, and thank God he's here in my lifetime.

"Katie has a long road ahead of her. We're kind of enjoying this time for this child and for Katie and my son as a family. There is going to come a time in the future when it's not going to be so easy. It's not going to be easy on Cal; it's not going to be easy for Katie or this child or us. We're celebrating right now, because this is something to celebrate."

One of Dr. Stelling's administrative staff interrupted Stelling and Hughes to remind them that they needed to leave and get ready for the Kokopelli Ball. "By the time you get home, the car is going to be there," she prodded.

The ball at Manhattan's Chelsea Piers was a who's who of reproductive doctors in the New York metropolitan area.

Tonight the society would be renamed; it would no longer be the American Infertility Association but the American Fertility Association, to focus on the positive rather than the negative.

Dara Torres, then a nine-time Olympic medal winner, had needed fertility help to get pregnant; she was a glamorous mistress of ceremonies, dressed in a sparkling blue-sequined dress. Brooke Shields, who'd needed fertility assistance to have her two daughters, was guest speaker.

Torres presented Dr. Howard Jones a lifetime award for the work he'd done with his wife, Dr. Georgeanna Jones. The two achieved the first IVF baby in the country in 1981. Howard Jones, who was ninety-two and had white hair, a cane, and a red flower in his lapel, walked slowly to the front of the room to accept the accolades. Dr. Hughes and the rest of the room gave him a standing ovation.

Then Torres introduced Shields. "I do like men, but I can't stop staring at her, she's even prettier in person," Torres said.

"You know, Dara," Shields sparred back, "because of the people in this room, you and me probably could have a baby together."

Everyone laughed.

————

Once the speakers were finished, the doctors mingled. "People who can get pregnant at home the fun way don't know anybody in this room," Hughes said. He was there to network with the doctors for whom his laboratory did PGD and to explain to other doctors what he did for couples and their embryos.

"So much of who we are happens at the beginning," Hughes said. "We have to look at that and understand that if we're going to understand the heartbreak that occurs if we don't pay any attention. After all, what is medicine? It's intercepting the normal course of disease, the natural course of Mother Nature. Whether we're giving a child a vaccine or we're delivering a baby by cesarean section so it has a chance to survive the birth or we're helping somebody to get pregnant, we're interrupting nature. One of the areas we have to focus on is at the beginning of life. At the turn of the century, the biggest killer of women was childbirth. We don't think of childbirth as being a life-threatening illness. When a woman gets pregnant, she doesn't think it might take her life. That's not even in the equation anymore. Why? Because medicine has interrupted nature. And that's good. If I give your child an antibiotic for an earache, I'm fooling around with Mother Nature. If I do open-heart surgery on a president, I'm interrupting the normal course of nature. I'm interested in genetic problems that occur at the beginning of life."

The beginning of life. Americans disagree over exactly when that is. That's one of the many reasons why preimplantation genetic diagnosis has stirred controversy and deeply troubles some bioethicists.

16

"It's Hard to Tell Parents, 'Don't Do This'"

Doctors have formed embryos outside the body for more than thirty years. But when parents use preimplantation genetic diagnosis to try to select a donor sibling, they are no longer choosing the embryo most likely to make a healthy baby. They are instead choosing the embryo they need to meet their goal of curing someone else. This application marked a shift in the use of PGD from a test employed purely to eliminate the chance of a disease or medical defect in a baby to one used to select a child with a preferred characteristic.

"I understand that a family could create, out of love, a new child [for the purpose of saving the life of a sibling]," said Alan Fleischman, a pediatrician and member of the New York State Task Force on Life and the Law. "We should not trivialize the pain families go through in making these decisions, or decide that they are being inappropriate, or that they don't really care, or that it's done without love for the new child. I would bet that anyone who spent time with a family in the throes of these problems would understand how hard this decision is, and how it's figured out with love and concern on the part of the family."

Many members of the medical community seem comfortable with using PGD to select a sibling who is a bone marrow match for a sick child. Some even go so far as to say there is a moral imperative to help a sick child if there is the medical means to accomplish it.

But, as with many procedures that involve the use of embryos, some ethicists and members of the general public become uncomfortable. Some ask how much influence we should wield at the beginning of life, whether the randomness of birth should be manipulated. Others ask how far we are willing to push the donor concept—who will balance the rights of the new child against the needs of the sick sibling, for example.

To begin with, the PGD process for donor selection can entail rejecting embryos that are perfectly viable; their only "flaw" is not matching the sick child. People who adamantly believe life begins at the joining of sperm and egg consider rejecting embryos wrong for any reason; no form of IVF will ever be acceptable to them based on the same principle. In any in vitro fertilization procedure—whether to help with infertility, to screen embryos for inherited disease, or to select an embryo as a tissue match for a sick sibling—more viable embryos are often produced than are needed to create a single baby. In those cases, the couple chooses what to do with the excess embryos: discard them, donate them to research or to another couple, or freeze them for possible future use in trying to have another child themselves. Fertility experts say many couples return to a reproductive endocrinologist to have another child and thaw out their frozen embryos to get pregnant. In those cases, freezing is advantageous, as getting pregnant with frozen embryos is less invasive and less expensive than undergoing another cycle of egg retrieval to create new embryos. But for couples who have had as many children as they want, the decision about what to do with frozen embryos hangs over them, sometimes for years. In the case of families who are seeking an HLA match, they may not be interested in freezing healthy embryos that aren't a match because they see no need for those embryos in their future.

In 2002, the national Society for Assisted Reproductive Technology surveyed the nation's 430 IVF clinics to get an idea of how many embryos were frozen in the United States. The estimate, garnered from the 340 clinics that responded: 400,000.

Jim Sedlak is vice president of the American Life League, a Virginia-based organization with a U.S. mailing list of 350,000; it opposes abortion and embryonic stem cell research. Sedlak believes the rejection of embryos for any reason—including that they can't help an ill sibling—is wrong.

"When an embryo dies, a human being dies," he insisted. "At fertilization, when the sperm and the egg join, the DNA is set at that point. Everything about that human being—how tall they are going to be, whether it will be male or female, the color of the eyes—all that is set at fertilization. Now you get to this variation where they do genetic testing and the human being has to pass a test in order to be allowed to pass on to the next phase of their life. We are totally opposed to that."

Even if an already-born child is saved by a donor child, that doesn't justify it, he said. "The emotions are with the child you can see and hold in your arms and photograph, as opposed to the children who are in the laboratory being conceived through in vitro fertilization and don't look like children to the average person."

Even doctors who don't believe rejecting an embryo involves the death of a human being are nonetheless sometimes uncomfortable producing healthy embryos they know won't be used. "While recognizing that clearly you can have excess embryos from many IVF cycles, the intent when we create those embryos is to create a baby," said Dr. David Adamson, director of Fertility Physicians of Northern California and president of the American Society for Reproductive Medicine from 2008 to 2009. The production of excess embryos is a residual effect of the intended act, which is to create a child. He sees that as morally different from making healthy embryos he knows he's not going to use to create a child. "If we create embryos that are healthy but aren't a match, the concern is what's going to happen to those," he said. They are more than just an insignificant by-product; they deserve to be treated with respect, he and other doctors believe. Adamson encourages his patients to donate excess embryos to research or to couples who want a child. His lab donates excess embryos to the University of California, San Francisco, for research. But some scientists note that in vitro fertilization with PGD reduces the numbers of abortions. Prior to the advent of PGD, desperate parents of children with the bone marrow disorder Fanconi anemia, for instance, were getting pregnant naturally and in some cases aborting if amniocentesis of the fetus showed it wasn't a tissue match for the ill sibling, said Arleen Auerbach, who runs the International Fanconi Anemia Registry at Rockefeller University in Manhattan.

"In my mind, that was the reason for doing this, to prevent abortions," said Dr. John Wagner from the University of Minnesota. In 2000, he helped the Nashes of Denver become the first family in the world to successfully select a donor sibling. "I was responding to what was happening in this patient community."

In England, where the Human Fertilisation and Embryology Authority has jurisdiction over reproductive matters, a distinction was initially made in granting permission to do PGD for sibling matching. The HFEA said yes to families who had already been planning to use PGD to make sure a future child didn't have an inherited disease that a sibling had and who decided they wanted to add on the testing that would determine if the healthy embryo could provide a bone marrow match. It said no to families who didn't need PGD to test for disease but were using it solely to make sure they had a donor match.

Here's why, experts said: pulling a cell off an embryo to do PGD to make sure an embryo didn't have an inherited disease offered a benefit to that embryo that outweighed any risk that might be involved. Since the family was pulling a cell off already anyway, they could add the HLA-matching test without incurring further risk to the embryo. However, in cases when the embryo was tested solely to see if it had the power to save its sibling's life, there was no gain for the embryo itself. The HFEA initially argued PGD hadn't been around long enough to ensure no long-term effects, and therefore it wasn't fair to have an embryo undergo a potentially risky biopsy for the benefit of someone else.

Denied British families traveled to the United States to have the PGD done. Under public pressure, England's authority later reversed itself and began to approve such use of PGD. European countries that regulate the use of reproductive technology have struggled with how to limit the use of PGD, and the complex regulations often change. "Each country has different rules," said Luca Gianaroli, chairman of the European Society of Human Reproduction and Embryology, an umbrella organization that is the European equivalent of the American Society for Reproductive Medicine. As of 2009, Italy, for instance, has specifically denied PGD for HLA matching, saying that even though the creation of a savior sibling may be a noble idea, a human being should never be the means to an end. It also doesn't allow PGD for fertile couples, making HLA matching a moot point, because couples with an ill child obviously aren't infertile, Gianaroli said. (There are no similar regulations in effect in the United States.)

Most of the information on the long-term health and well-being of the savior or donor siblings in the United States is anecdotal, gleaned from doctors or geneticists who follow up with families; they say they have not seen any abnormalities.

A study done in Belgium of 583 children born after PGD done for various reasons showed that they didn't have any more major health effects than children born after assisted reproductive technologies that didn't include PGD. No specific defect has been consistently found in any report, said Joe Leigh Simpson, who monitored such information in his role as president of the Preimplantation Genetic Diagnosis International Society from 2007 to 2009. The rate of birth defects seems to be 2 to 3 percent, he said. "It appears to be the same as the general population and not worth losing sleep over." He admitted that the number of children monitored was small and that the oldest child conceived by PGD was born in 1990 and is still young.

While there may be no direct benefit for the donor child, the family as a whole benefits, and that makes the choice morally acceptable, some bioethicists argue. "You're doing something that is not for the benefit of the younger sibling but is not harming them," said

Auerbach, who routinely interacts with families of Fanconi anemia patients. "They wouldn't have been born otherwise, and meanwhile they are helping the family unit, including parents, grandparents, and any existing normal siblings."

In addition to the controversy about what should or shouldn't be done to embryos, there is the concern of some doctors and ethicists about the health of the expectant mother and the implanted embryos. Might reproductive endocrinologists take medical chances, going to greater lengths to get a woman pregnant because they are racing the clock to save a sick child? Might they implant too many embryos, creating triplets or more, which could be a risk to the children sharing the womb and to the mother? Because no one is following the use of PGD for HLA matching, whether these concerns are hypothetical or real isn't known. "I try not to ask myself questions beyond this: if you can cure disease and not harm the child conceived in the process, if the family is going to love that child just like any other child, then I think it's fine to do it," said Dr. Jeffrey Lipton, Katie's Diamond Blackfan anemia doctor. "You talk to a parent striving for their child to live to their next birthday, to get to Christmas, it's hard to tell parents, 'Don't do this.'"

When Katie's parents considered creating a sibling, they had few other families to seek out for advice—the two geneticists who perform most of the tissue matching in the United States estimated that prior to 2006 only between 100 and 200 such donor children existed worldwide. The number has now climbed to about 250, according to the experts' estimates. Mark Hughes said that as of 2009 he had performed PGD for tissue matching that had resulted in 162 births. According to numbers reported by the Preimplantation Genetic Diagnosis International Society at the group's conference in Miami in April of 2009, Chicago's Reproductive Genetics Institute, the laboratory of Dr. Yury Verlinsky, had reported the births of 50 donor siblings. About 30 more had been born in Europe, according to Gianaroli of the European Society of Human Reproduction and Embryology. About 1,000 families had attempted IVF with PGD to select a donor sibling, said Anver Kuliev, who works at Verlinsky's practice in Chicago and was executive director of the society. (Dr. Verlinsky died of colon cancer on July 16, 2009, at the age of sixty-five.)

The scientists who perform PGD are fertility and genetics specialists, and different teams of experts do the subsequent bone marrow transplants, so nobody knows how many siblings actually provide transplants or how many have been successful. No person or organization in the United States is known to be collecting data on which choice doctors are more frequently making: umbilical-cord blood or marrow extraction from the new child. Dr. Vlachos, using the Diamond Blackfan Anemia Registry at Schneider Children's Hospital, is trying to quantify the prevalence and success rates for umbilical-cord versus bone marrow transplants for DBA patients, even though the registry wasn't initially intended to compile this data. Despite all the attention paid to the subject of savior siblings, there simply aren't any reliable statistics regarding how many are born each year, how many donate cord blood or bone marrow or both, and how often those transplants are successful.

According to the small amount of savior-sibling data that was voluntarily collected from U.S. fertility doctors for the first time in 2006 by the Genetics and Public Policy Center at Johns Hopkins University in Washington, D.C., sibling matching accounts for about 1 percent of all PGD cycles. The rest of the time PGD is used to test embryos for inherited diseases or for chromosomal abnormalities. Of three thousand PGD cycles reported in 2005, forty-three were for donor matching, said Susannah Baruch, director of law and policy at the center. (A PGD cycle is defined as each time a woman uses PGD to try to get pregnant during one menstrual cycle. If she fails to get pregnant and has to try again the following month, that counts as a separate PGD cycle.) The questionnaire didn't ask whether any babies were actually born after those cycles, Baruch said. It's estimated that ten thousand children worldwide have been born using PGD, but no American organization has tallied these births, and Hughes said the numbers are guesses at best. "It could be on the low side, but if it's low, it's low by one or two thousand," said Joe Leigh Simpson of the PGD International Society.

Scientists involved with PGD for sibling matching say they'd like to know the success rate of producing donor children, how many subsequent transplants are done with cord blood versus bone marrow, how often transplants succeed, how many times in the future a donor child is called upon to aid the sibling, and how often, if at all, PGD children experience future physical or psychological problems.

The Society for Assisted Reproductive Technology (SART) has begun to ask American fertility clinics how often PGD is being used and for what purposes. But it's far from a full-fledged registry. That would take a commitment of a great sum of money to fund the project, collect the data, and follow the children as they grow up, said Dr. Elizabeth Ginsburg, president of SART from 2008 to 2009. According to the latest data collected by the organization, U.S. fertility clinics reported doing 9,032 PGD cycles in 2007. The birth rate was slightly higher than 26 percent, meaning about 2,350 babies were born after those cycles, Ginsburg said. The statistics didn't break down the number of cycles done for bone marrow tissue matching, but the number was "really small," Ginsburg said.

A registry of PGD offspring is the least that should be done, and it should be sure to place children conceived as donors in their own category, said George Annas, head of the department of Health Law, Bioethics, and Human Rights at Boston University. "So we can say in ten years, 'Is this good for kids, or is this bad for kids?' I'm not saying I'm against it, but I'm in favor of keeping statistics on it and protecting the child—the donor—from exploitation."

The moral and ethical issues surrounding the selection of a donor sibling don't end with the baby's birth. That donor sibling assumes a unique role in the life of the sick child and the entire family. A perfect match for life, this child could be called upon should the sick sibling have additional medical needs. Parents who would normally make medical decisions in the best interests of their baby will have to advocate for two children whose interests may diverge.

While some ethicists say they are okay with the umbilical-cord blood and even actual bone marrow being used to provide a sick sibling with a transplant, they fear that may not be where the demands on the donor sibling end. They ask: what if the parents need the donor child again, only this time it's for, say, a kidney for the sibling? While children who are coincidental matches for their ill siblings—such as Keir Zangrando's sister, Emma—also have parents who are deciding for two children, some ethicists worry that parents who have purposely conceived donor children might be quicker to call upon that child whenever necessary.

17

"There's No Black-and-White Answer"

Once a donor child is born, decisions about his or her health and body are made by the parents. "I'm concerned with the real, live children," said George Annas, head of the department of Health Law, Bioethics, and Human Rights at Boston University. "That's what you have to be concerned with—the embryos that go on to become children. The first issue is whether you're having a baby just to be a donor. All parents deny that. They've learned the right answer to that question."

Beyond that, there's the issue of how the donor child is used to help his or her sibling, Annas said. For example, if the cord blood from the donor child isn't enough to save the sibling, doctors then go to that child for bone marrow, extracting it from the back of the child's hips in an operating room, inserting a needle numerous times into each hip. This can be a painful procedure and has its own risks to the donor, such as infection and adverse reactions to anesthesia. To Annas, going beyond the cord blood crosses the line. If bone marrow is taken, he says, "Then the question is, 'How often do you have to do this?' Hopefully it's just once."

Jeffrey Kahn, director of the Center for Bioethics at the University of Minnesota, shares Annas's concerns. "When you take a one-year-old to the OR, presumably under general anesthesia, and you stick a big old needle in his hip, you have to think about how much risk you are willing to take," Kahn said. "How far up the level of risk would you expose the healthy child for therapeutic treatment for the sick child?"

Beyond the parents and the doctors of the ill sibling, there is nobody looking at the rights of the donor child. "There is nobody equipped to say, 'Hold your horses. Wait a second. Let's look at what's going on with the donor child,'" said Kahn's colleague Susan Wolf, a professor of law, medicine, and public policy at the University of Minnesota. "This is a living, feeling human being with his or her own interests. How many times would you have gone to the hospital for your brother or sister, been anesthetized, and submitted to a bone marrow harvest? The answer to that would vary depending on each child and each family. A kid may not really want to play that role. If you were dealing with a ten-year-old, you might see something very disturbing. You might see a ten-year-old freaking out. A baby isn't capable of mounting protest."

While a parent—in theory, at least—would do anything to save his or her child, a sibling might not. Sometimes hospitals will pass cases by an ethical review board, but it's not required.

Some ethicists also worry about the mental health of the donor child down the road, once he or she learns the history of the conception. "The parents are going to have to communicate to the child that the child is valued for his or her own characteristics and life, in addition to being created to save his sibling," said Adrienne Asch, who teaches bioethics at Yeshiva University in New York City. "In the same way that children can resent one another for all kinds of things, or can be jealous of each other or feel that they are not as valued by a parent, you obviously have plenty of potential sibling problems here. There's no way out of that. That doesn't mean the parents shouldn't do this, but they better be aware of what they are doing."

What the child may later feel is a matter of speculation, said Elizabeth Grill, psychologist at the Center for Reproductive Medicine and Infertility at New York–Presbyterian/Weill Cornell Medical Center in Manhattan. She counsels couples undergoing PGD. "There's no black-and-white answer, because it really depends on the family dynamics and the evaluation of each family," she said.

If the transplant succeeds, and the donor child is elevated to hero status, she said, this could lead to a special role in the family that could be either easy or difficult to handle. "On the one hand, the children could feel an incredible closeness to each other," Grill said. "On the other hand, there could be these conflicted feelings of 'I feel used,' or 'I don't have a choice.'" In addition to the donor child having issues, the recipient could also feel guilty or grateful. "We see this with sister donations of eggs. The recipient feels like they can never possibly repay this. What can you possibly give to repay the gift of life?"

And what if the transplant from the donor child fails? "If a child is born and the older sibling dies, what will that do to the donor child?" asked Thomas Murray, president of the Hastings Center in Garrison, New York, a research institute devoted to ethical issues in medicine and the life sciences. Will the child feel he failed in the role he was born to play? "I think that would be a challenge to parent," Murray said. "I'm not a person who believes that life is neat and tidy and runs smoothly. I can imagine strong families surviving that challenge very well. I could imagine others not so well."

In 2004, Jodi Picoult, a best-selling author who coincidentally grew up in the same Long Island community the Trebings live in and attended the same high school as Stacy Trebing, published a novel called *My Sister's Keeper* to explore such emotional issues. In it she created a scenario in which a thirteen-year-old savior sister created through in vitro fertilization and preimplantation genetic diagnosis sued her family so she wouldn't have to continue propping up her older sister's health, this time with a kidney transplant. The book was a best seller and became a major motion picture; it was released in June of 2009 and starred Alec Baldwin, Cameron Diaz, and Abigail Breslin. Clearly the subject was very compelling to American readers and moviegoers. But because the oldest documented donor child worldwide is not yet thirteen, such a scenario couldn't yet happen.

Picoult wanted to explore the worst-case scenario—that a donor child's cord blood or onetime bone marrow transplant wasn't enough. That the sick child who was supposed to be saved actually got sicker, and needed more help from the donor sibling. "I needed to ratchet up the stakes a little. I really tried to create a situation and a disease burden that would require Anna, the donor child, to donate frequently, sometimes with methods that were very invasive, so that she was tapped multiple times to save her sister. And that changes the situation considerably," Picoult said. "I really spun the story out in several directions. The first being 'What will happen when a donor child becomes a teenager?' Teenagers are always thinking about themselves and who they are and who they want to be. Will a donor child be wondering, 'Gee, would I even be here if my sister wasn't sick?'"

Stacy Trebing's former high-school biology teacher, who served with Stacy on the local blood bank's advisory board, told Stacy about the book that Picoult, also his former student, had written. Stacy said she started reading *My Sister's Keeper* while she was pregnant with Katie's donor sibling but couldn't finish it. It was too emotionally upsetting, especially since, in another coincidence, the sick child was named Kate.

When Picoult wrote the book, she talked to the pioneering Nash family. Lisa and Jack Nash of Englewood, Colorado, said they used PGD to find an embryo that didn't have the bone marrow disorder Fanconi anemia and also would be a bone marrow match for their daughter Molly. The Nashes speak to reporters from all over the world about what they did to cure their daughter. "By us being public, other people learn about it," Lisa Nash said.

Fanconi anemia is similar to Diamond Blackfan anemia in that the patient needs regular blood transfusions to stay alive. In 2000, Molly was a few months from death when she had her bone marrow transplant using blood from Adam's umbilical cord, Lisa Nash said. "The spark had died. She couldn't walk, people had to carry her," Lisa said. Molly loved to dance but didn't have the energy. Her dance teacher would say to her, "Dance with me." Molly would reply, "No, you dance, and I'll watch you."

Saving Molly's life was not the sole reason the Nashes had Adam, Lisa Nash said. "We had Adam first and foremost because we wanted a bigger family," she said. The Nashes said they would have had Adam through PGD to ensure he didn't have Fanconi anemia even if they hadn't had the option of also checking for sibling matching. "The fact that he was able to help her really was icing on the cake."

Molly had a bone marrow transplant using Adam's umbilical-cord blood the month after he was born. Her bone marrow is now free of Fanconi anemia. However, there are still concerns about her health. "These kids are still very prone to certain types of cancer. We watch her very closely for head and neck cancers," said Lisa Nash. Molly has other physical ailments related to her disease. She is deaf in one ear, was born without thumbs, and is fed with a feeding tube. Her thyroid failed—a late-term effect of the chemotherapy that preceded the cord-blood transplant—and she has also had surgery to correct cataracts.

But Molly is a teenager now. "The spirit in her and the fire in her—she is just an amazing, amazing kiddo," her mother said. The Nashes have since had another child, Delaine, who was also born using PGD to avoid Fanconi anemia.

The Nashes said they don't talk to the children about the role Adam played in Molly's survival. "If you asked Adam what happened, he'd say, 'I gave Molly my blood so she would feel better.' Someday when they're old enough, we'll explain it to them," Lisa Nash said. "We want our kids to have normal lives and be just like everybody else." She scoffs at critics who fret that donor children such as Adam might one day feel they weren't really wanted. "Adam, being the sole male [child] in the family, he is the be-all and end-all," she said. "The ethicists, that's their job, to doubt everything everybody does and to raise questions. I guarantee you if any ethicist spent time with us they would change what they are saying."

To anyone who worries taking a cell from an embryo—as is done in PGD testing—might prove harmful later, Lisa Nash said of her son, "He walks and he talks and he reads. The only thing we see is he can't play basketball, but neither can his father. If you want to attribute something to pulling off the single cell, he can't play basketball."

As for how much they would use Adam in the future to help Molly, Lisa Nash said she and her husband decided before Adam was born they would only use his cord blood, not his bone marrow, to cure Molly. "Adam was brought here because we loved Adam and not for spare parts," she said. The cord blood, she said, was "his garbage. He didn't need it anymore. When it came to taking bone marrow from Adam, that wasn't okay in our eyes. That's where we drew the line." So far, they haven't had to test their resolve.

Lisa Nash won't judge other people who might make different decisions. "I think people need to be really cautious about judging people. Until you have a sick child and you watch your child suffer, you don't really know what you would do. Be thankful you have healthy kids and don't have to agonize over these decisions."

Nash said she is a proponent of government oversight of the use of PGD technology. "The government should look at it and put some kind of boundaries and barriers," she said. If the technology was regulated, she said, insurance companies might pay for the procedures. She said she and her husband spent $250,000 to have Adam because they had to go through in vitro fertilization five times before it worked. They took out a loan to pay for it.

Marissa Ayala, whose parents conceived her naturally, hoping she would be a bone marrow match for her older sister, Anissa, doesn't usually talk publicly about her story. But in 2009, when Marissa was eighteen, an essay appeared in *Teen Vogue*—her story as told to writer Angela Wu. In it, she said:

> I first started really researching my own story when I was in the seventh grade. My friends were Googling themselves and nothing came up, but when I searched for myself a lot of news articles popped up. I read negative comments from

a few newspapers about how my parents were just using me to save my sister's life and weren't going to love me, and that what they did was morally wrong. It surprised me. I thought, "Really? People think about my family like that?" Some of the articles said that if I hadn't been a perfect match for my sister, my parents would have disowned me. And that just wasn't the case.

I try to see both sides of the story, but I ultimately don't agree with the critics. They were probably just looking out for my safety, thinking that my parents were going to have a baby solely for the purpose of saving their child. But they don't know us personally: My family loves me so much.

That's also what Picoult said she found when she did the research for *My Sister's Keeper*. "A lot of the parents I spoke to when I did my research really love these children so much because they're heroes in their families. They're little tiny superheroes. They saved someone's life. I have yet to meet a family that has become involved in this situation that hasn't desperately wanted another child in the family and loved them even more for being able to save the sibling's life.

"If I were the mother of a child who had leukemia, and that child needed a bone marrow transplant, I would not hesitate in using PGD to try to create an embryo that would be a donor match. I know I would do it. Creating a donor sibling is not eugenics because you are not looking for a higher IQ, you're not looking for a blond baby, you're not even looking for a girl or a boy. What you're looking for are six HLA proteins that nobody in their right mind would even care about if they weren't trying to give a donation of bone marrow. It's a match in a way that doesn't matter to anyone except the person doing the transplant.

"Of course the 'slippery slope' is that, if you can manipulate these six HLA proteins, eventually we'll be able to manipulate intelligence and emotion, popularity and good looks and athletic ability, and that's where it becomes dangerous. These parents are not asking for something that anyone would consider to be a characteristic that is in some way trying to create a master race, or even a more gifted child."

But critics worry that it's only a matter of time before some parents will ask for just that.

18

"We're Not Going to Stop the Future"

Over the next few generations, the use of preimplantation genetic diagnosis and preimplantation genetic screening may become as common as amniocentesis, predicts David Adamson, a past president of the American Society for Reproductive Medicine. Doctors could ensure a healthy embryo, extending life spans to ninety, Adamson said. "This is a technology that's increasingly going to redefine health care," he said. "It's going to determine how babies are born, and how we re-create ourselves."

Other reproductive endocrinologists echo Adamson. "The technology is moving along," said Dr. Daniel Kenigsberg, who directs a thriving IVF clinic on Long Island. "We're probably within five years of screening hundreds of genes on any given embryo. There is the possibility that IVF could become the treatment of the fertile as opposed to the treatment of the infertile. That may actually be a positive thing."

While PGD was originally meant to avoid life-threatening hereditary diseases that appear in childhood, some parents are already screening embryos for gene mutations that may give a child the tendency to develop a disease much later in life, such as breast cancer. PGD is now also being used to avoid afflictions that aren't fatal, such as an eye condition that could lead to blindness. PGD pioneer Mark Hughes is comfortable with families trying to eliminate such diseases from their descendants. "No one understands these diseases better than the family who has it," he said. "We can sit around a mahogany table and debate this, but this family lives with the disease every day and knows it's serious enough to go through such extraordinary approaches to avoid giving it to the next generation."

A variation of PGD, now frequently referred to as preimplantation genetic screening, or PGS, allows scientists to screen for chromosomal abnormalities, such as Down syndrome. Doctors such as PGD pioneer Alan Handyside are now working on new techniques to assess embryos, such as karyomapping, which looks at one embryonic cell's entire genome of inheritance from the parents.

Julian Savulescu, who is a professor of ethics at St. Cross College in Oxford, coined a term for choosing the best embryo—*procreative beneficence*—suggesting that if a couple has the ability to produce the healthiest child, they have a moral obligation to do so. Savulescu argued in the publication *Bioethics* that "couples should select embryos or fetuses which are most likely to have the best life, based on available genetic information, including information about non-disease genes." By *non-disease genes* he means genes for characteristics such as height, intelligence, and character.

While doctors such as Adamson and Hughes see the good in testing embryos for the avoidance of disease, others are chilled by what they see as potential abuse of the process. They point out that one day scientists may be able to pinpoint genes for such nonmedical traits as Savulescu mentioned—and also characteristics that are purely preference, such as hair color or complexion. So while parents tested for Alzheimer's or cancer genes, they would also have the ability to test for favored eye color or, perhaps, musical ability. The science may move from guaranteeing a healthy baby free of certain diseases to customizing the child, choosing the embryo that will have certain traits the parents desire.

"Will parents try to do that? Really select a child's characteristics the way you can pick the options on a car?" asked Thomas Murray, president of the Hastings Center, a research institute in New York State devoted to ethical issues. "Not many. But it doesn't take many to make it an issue." Already one doctor in California has advertised that his clinic could offer parents some choice in a baby's eye color and skin color. He posted the advertisement on his clinic's Web site in March of 2009, though he swiftly rescinded the advertising after it created a media uproar and backlash from fellow doctors.

Parents could one day end up engaging in "micro-eugenics," said Stanford University physician and bioethicist William Hurlbut, who served as a member of George W. Bush's President's Council on Bioethics. Rather than a state-imposed program of eugenics, the parents themselves might one by one weed out genes they considered undesirable, he said. "Someone could easily make the argument that being short is like a disease because it may result in social disadvantages," Hurlbut said. He pointed out that more complex traits, such as intelligence, will be far harder to select for because they depend on the interaction of many genes.

Prospective parents could potentially try to weed out characteristics such as homosexuality, if that is found to be a genetic trait, as some scientists have argued it is. "Many people wouldn't want to have a child with that trait," said one bioethicist who didn't want to be named.

And there is also the possibility that parents could choose a trait that most of the population might find undesirable. There has already been one set of lesbian deaf parents who wanted to conceive a deaf child and so intentionally sought out a deaf sperm donor. In 2002, Sharon Duchesneau and Candy McCullough, both of whom had been born deaf, requested a deaf sperm donor from clinics and were turned down. They then enlisted a deaf friend to help them conceive because they viewed deafness not as a disability but as a culture, and they wanted their future child to share it with them.

As there are no regulations or laws about how PGD can be used in the United States, it is up to individual doctors and hospital administrators to decide whether they will perform PGD for nonmedical reasons.

"Responsible physicians hopefully will not perform PGD for frivolous reasons," said Zev Rosenwaks, director of the Center for Reproductive Medicine and Infertility at New York–Presbyterian/Weill Cornell Medical Center in Manhattan. "The theoretical applications of PGD are essentially in the science fiction realm. PGD is here to alleviate pain and suffering. If one follows that tenet, it is a relatively simple thing to follow." Prior to PGD, families with a history of, say, Huntington's disease often did not have children for fear of passing it on, Rosenwaks said. His clinic does three hundred PGD cycles per year, primarily to test for genetic and chromosomal abnormalities. He will not do embryo selection for nonmedical reasons, he said.

Neither would Kuliev and Verlinsky's clinic in Chicago. "We have done more than five thousand cases," Kuliev said. "We have never had a request to do something stupid like selecting something unethical. Those who are talking about ethical issues, they are probably not involved in the medical profession. We are not selecting the color of the eyes, and nobody has ever requested us to do so."

Many scientists support doctors being the gatekeepers for PGD usage, rather than, as in England, a regulatory panel. "Like most of the things in medical practice, you don't have to have permission before you do anything," said John Robertson, an ethicist at the University of Texas. The government doesn't regulate choosing cosmetic surgery, for instance. "People often say we need that for PGD, but why?"

For his part, Adamson argues that widespread use of PGD testing should be implemented carefully. "There's so much fearmongering that goes on about everything. I think the technology has a lot of potential. I think we have to implement this very carefully, and we need a lot of social input. We don't want to throw it out because people worry about a slippery slope. If the outcome is a healthy baby for, let's call it, ninety years, was it worth the IVF? I think so. I think so. I don't live in fear of the future. I think we have to be confident in ourselves as a people and as a nation, that we will face these things. Let's weed the bad out as we come to it. We're not going to stop the future, and we're not going to stop the technology."

Some experts keeping an eye on PGD research, such as Francis Fukuyama, a professor at the Johns Hopkins School of Advanced International Studies, in Washington, D.C., call for a new arm of government to oversee reproductive developments and breakthroughs. "We need a mechanism for determining the moral acceptability of new biomedical technologies that really reflects an informed, democratic discussion," said Fukuyama, a former member of President Bush's Council on Bioethics. "The scientists by themselves are not in a position to make those kinds of judgments."

He's under no illusion that that will happen soon. "What it's going to take is some accident or some cloning experiment that goes wrong for people to sit up and say, 'My God, I didn't know we could do these kinds of things,'" he said. "That's how regulation institutions have been created in this country, through some kind of crisis or accident."

Sean Tipton, spokesman for the American Society for Reproductive Medicine, called the idea of a new arm of government to regulate reproductive technologies a fantasy. "Americans tend not to want to have government making the decision about who gets to have kids and how and why," he said. "We think these decisions are best left up to the individuals."

Bioethicist Murray agreed: "The first option shouldn't be the heavy boot of the state." But there should be a public discussion of what it means to be a parent and how much control over the child's characteristics is healthy for the parent or child or society, Murray and others said.

"It does always seem to be valuable to try to reflect on how all of our individual choices are going to add up to new social forces, and understand whether these social forces are good ones or not," said Erik Parens, a senior research scholar and a colleague of Murray's at the Hastings Center. He said he worries about "genetic privilege."

"It strikes me as implausible that we're going to get from today, where almost fifty million people in the United States are without health care, to a world where everybody has access to PGD," Parens said. "There's no doubt in my mind that in a hundred years, people who already are privileged will have the privilege of using technologies like PGD."

Parens said he believes some sort of regulatory body is in order, to determine what is acceptable to do to an embryo and what is not. But he said that few politicians would want to tackle it. "As soon as you talk about doing things with embryos, you're immediately sucked into the abortion debate. It doesn't seem that with President Obama our conversation is getting less heated or otherwise clearer. The disagreement seems as rancorous as ever," Parens said. "It is a shame that because of the passion on the two sides of the abortion issue, we don't have an opportunity to have an open and clear debate about the difference between what we take to be reasonable things to do to embryos and what we take to be unreasonable things to do to embryos."

Marcy Darnovsky, the associate director of the Center for Genetics and Society, a public interest organization based in Oakland, California, that advocates the responsible use of genetic technology, said that left unregulated, the fertility industry could begin to push PGD aggressively for marketing reasons. "It's uncomfortable to think of anything related to a child and reproduction as an industry, but it has become a multibillion dollar technology," she said of IVF in all its uses. Half jokingly, she said doctors may begin to advertise, with slogans like "We give you an 82 percent chance of scoring 100 points higher on your SATs."

"The dangers are that under the pressure of marketing, parents will feel we have to do it to give our kids the best start in life," she said. "Then you set up this vicious cycle where people are seeking the perfect child. We lose a lot of what it means to be human in that and could find ourselves heading toward a world of genetic castes."

The 1997 science fiction movie *Gattaca* imagined such a world.

In the movie, middle- and upper-class parents routinely use technology to produce genetically superior babies. Children's DNA are analyzed, and based on the results, their places in life are determined, with more opportunities going to genetically superior humans. Vincent Freeman, played by Ethan Hawke, was conceived naturally and is born with a congenital heart defect that gives him a life expectancy of thirty years. He fights against the world that has relegated him to a menial labor job; it's his dream to be an astronaut. He borrows DNA from another man to try to outwit the system and get a job at the Gattaca aerospace company, and he lives in constant fear of being discovered for this illegal act.

In the real world, there are already nonmedical uses of PGD, such as gender selection purely for preference, that trouble some ethicists and scientists. Adamson said he was surprised by the results of a 2006 survey conducted by the Genetics and Public Policy Center at Johns Hopkins University which showed that close to half the PGD clinics that responded were offering to do gender selection for nonmedical reasons. It wasn't clear in the survey whether gender selection was allowed only when embryos were already being tested for disease. "Frankly, I was surprised that it was that high," he said. "There appears to be some real demand for this from people." Experts in the United States say that the trend in gender selection is to choose girls.

In June of 2004, the same month the Trebings were going through their rounds of PGD, a woman named Sharla Miller, a thirty-four-year-old from Wyoming, gave birth to twin girls, Brynne and Brooke. They were conceived with the help of a California reproductive endocrinologist who did PGD for her for what's been called "family balancing"—simply because Miller had already had three boys and wanted her next child to be a daughter.

Miller said she loved her sons enormously and attended every football practice and wrestling match and soccer game. But they were boys. "They fish and hunt and do all that stuff with their dad," Miller said. "I go along, not necessarily enjoying it, but to be part of the family. I just couldn't get it out of my system that I wanted a daughter. I just felt that our chances were slim to none. I could end up with twenty-five sons and not one daughter."

Gender-determination message boards on the Internet, where women emote about their quests to influence the sex of their next-borns, are filled with women who agree with Miller; the writers have user names such as Boysrus, Haveblue, and Prayingforpink. Ethicists worry about how those girls will be treated by their parents when they want to play with frogs and climb trees instead of wear pink dresses and paint their fingernails.

Right now, women who want to use PGD must go through IVF. Some feel that is a big enough barrier to deter women from using it for nonmedical reasons. Adamson isn't so sure, especially as IVF technology advances and becomes less invasive and onerous. For instance, some doctors are now using lower doses of ovarian stimulation medication or no medication, Adamson said, and others are experimenting with maturing eggs outside the body.

Currently, finding a reproductive endocrinologist who will do PGD solely for gender selection is not easy. The major medical societies have discouraged it. The use of PGD for gender selection is so controversial it's been banned in some countries, including England. PGD pioneer Hughes is "distressed" PGD is being used for anything other than medical reasons. "We think it is a misuse of medical technology," he said. Some doctors avoid elective PGD because they are worried about increased scrutiny from regulatory agencies or because they don't want to buck their medical association's recommendations. Others worry about how society as a whole will react. "If the field doesn't restrain itself, there's going to be some really ugly stuff down the line," said Dr. Daniel Kenigsberg, a Long Island reproductive endocrinologist. "At some point the technology can get ahead of society. Then at some point you are risking a backlash."

But an American couple who wants to pursue family balancing through PGD can certainly find a way. Dr. Richard Scott of Reproductive Medicine Associates in Morristown, New Jersey, a widely respected member of the American Fertility Association, began offering PGD to all patients in 2003 and has done about twenty to thirty purely for gender selection. At first, Scott had refused to do PGD for gender selection if the patient didn't already need fertility help. Then, one of his patients who already had two boys and wanted a girl asked Scott for IVF and PGD; he refused because she was perfectly fertile, so she had her tubes tied so that she would be a candidate for IVF. When she returned to Scott and announced that she now needed fertility help and asked again for PGD to have a girl, he was shocked.

"I nearly fell off my chair," he said. He said he felt "like a bad guy" because she'd undergone an unnecessary medical procedure. She'd taught him a lesson: patients will find ways around restrictions. He began to open the door but insisted his patients were counseled about the risks and costs. In vitro doesn't always work, and when it does, it can result in twins or triplets. Some cycles, women don't produce enough eggs to make it cost effective to add PGD. IVF costs between $8,000 and $14,000 per try, and PGD adds about $2,500 to $3,500. Insurance won't cover IVF for fertile people, and most companies don't even cover it entirely for infertile people. The Millers, for instance, spent $18,480 for the PGD procedure itself and about $7,000 for airfare, lodging, and fertility medication. "People have the right of self-determination. This is America," Scott said. "Well-counseled patients are grown-ups. They get to make decisions about their lives."

But could the United States one day wind up in a predicament similar to China's? Recent reports from that country predict that within fifteen years, China will have thirty million more men than women of marriageable age. This is the result of the Chinese government's restriction of one child per family, begun in 1979 and still officially in effect. Because the cultural preference for a male child is so strong there, some women choose to abort if prenatal testing shows the fetus is female.

Dr. Jeffrey Steinberg of the Fertility Institutes in Los Angeles, Manhattan, and Guadalajara, Mexico, openly advertises PGD for gender selection. He did the Millers' procedures, and he said he has treated about 5,000 other women, resulting in about 3,800 babies. "I didn't go into this thinking I was going to be a trailblazer, but I'm starting to think I am," he said.

In more areas than just elective gender selection. Steinberg was the doctor who in March of 2009 advertised the use of PGD to select for eye color or skin complexion. He posted a notice on his Fertility Institutes Web site that said this: *Predictive Genomics to be Available: Eye color, hair color, cancer tendency and more. New!*

The ad continued:

> We are pleased to announce the pending availability of a greatly expanded panel of available genetic tests that may be combined with our world-renowned aneuploidy [abnormal number of chromosomes] and gender selection testing. For the first time ever, patients having genetic screening for abnormal chromosome conditions in their embryos will be able to elect expanded testing that can greatly increase the odds of achieving a healthy pregnancy with a pre-selected choice of gender, eye color, hair color and complexion, along with the screening for potentially lethal diseases, screening for cancer tendencies (breast, colon, pancreas, prostate) and more.

An asterisk warned that limitations applied. For one thing, at that point, Steinberg could only help couples of Scandinavian descent choose their babies' eye color, because that population was geographically isolated enough to have primarily bred with other Scandinavians, making it easier to more precisely define the genes affecting their eye color. He would be able to tell them that one embryo had an 80 percent chance of green eyes, another a 40 percent chance, another a 10 percent chance. Also, the couples would be able to work only with the genes they had. "If they want brown eyes, and there's no brown eyes there, I can't make that happen," Steinberg said.

And clearly there's a market for selecting traits that have nothing to do with health. Dr. Mark Hughes tells of a team of Asian businessmen who once approached him to start a business in Japan that would offer Japanese parents children with more Western-shaped eyes. (The businessmen didn't understand until Hughes explained it to them: if the parents didn't have the genes for a characteristic, their children couldn't have that characteristic.)

Steinberg's bold advertisement drew the ire of Marcy Darnovsky's Center for Genetics and Society, which issued a press release to the media nationwide: *This development, along with the birth of octuplets to a Southern California woman* [Nadya Suleman, who gave birth in January of 2009], *brings new attention to the urgent need for effective regulation and oversight of the multi-billion dollar assisted reproduction industry in the U.S.,* it said. *Assisted reproduction in America has been a Wild West for too long. Responsible oversight of extreme reproductive technologies such as embryo selection based on skin color is long overdue.*

The media covered the controversy, declaring that the age of designer babies had arrived, and Steinberg was vilified by critics. He withdrew his advertisement, saying it wasn't worth the heat to continue to offer elective selection of traits at that point. "That was a misstep," Steinberg said of his foray into selection for nonmedical traits. He thinks he was just too premature in introducing the concept to the public. But he believes it will come up again, maybe ten years from now. "I'm happy we at least got it out there," he said. He plans to use selection of eye color or skin color to help people medically to avoid albinism or a family history of melanoma. But before he offers elective trait selection again, he will consult with ethicists, he said.

Adamson points out that Steinberg was reined in by public pressure that, as he'd predicted, weeded out an undesirable use of PGD. "This is an example where society said, 'We don't agree with this and we don't accept this. This may be available, but this is not the right thing to do.'"

19

"It's a Boy!"

"It's a boy!" Dr. Brian McKenna declared on May 4, 2005, when Christopher Thomas Trebing entered the world.

At seven o'clock that morning, just over one year after the Trebings began their quest to have a third child, Stacy Trebing walked into St. Catherine of Siena Medical Center in nearby Smithtown to deliver her baby. She wasn't having contractions, and the baby wasn't due for another week. But because of the crucial importance of collecting the umbilical-cord blood, as well as the size of the baby, Stacy had been scheduled to be induced.

The staff had started Stacy on a Pitocin IV drip to jump-start contractions, and a few hours later, McKenna, Stacy's obstetrician, inserted an instrument into Stacy's uterus to break her water. Warm liquid gushed out, and Stacy could feel her belly deflating. She asked for a painkilling epidural.

Everything was normal.

Stacy's parents were permitted in the labor room with Steve, and the four chatted and shared orange-flavored ice chips, the only food Stacy was allowed. At three thirty, a nurse checked on Stacy, saw she was fully dilated and almost ready to push, and asked her parents to leave the room.

Steve put on latex gloves, but he was too nervous to participate in the birth process. "Do you want to feel the head?" Dr. McKenna asked.

"No," Steve said.

"Come on, the head is right there," McKenna encouraged.

Still, Steve declined. He didn't want to do anything that might jinx the delivery and the collection of the cord blood.

Stacy had a hard time pushing. At one point, the baby was twisting and McKenna had to align the fetus. Stacy thought Steve was going to faint.

Still, everything proceeded normally, and Christopher finally slid into the room at five o'clock that evening. Tipping the scales at nine pounds, one ounce, he was the biggest of the three Trebing children.

"Is he okay?" Stacy asked. "Does everything look good?"

"Yes," McKenna said.

Steve thought Christopher looked a shade of blue. McKenna placed Christopher on Stacy's stomach.

"Do you want to cut the umbilical cord?" McKenna asked Steve.

"No," Steve answered, still afraid.

McKenna snipped it. He held the severed cord and extracted its blood—the life force they all hoped would conquer Katie's Diamond Blackfan anemia. It filled a heavy plastic collection bag.

"This is great!" McKenna said. "You're going to have a big bag. One of the biggest collections I've ever seen."

"Is he a good color?" Stacy asked about Christopher. She was thinking, *Not pale, indicating Diamond Blackfan anemia?*

"Yes," McKenna assured her. Stacy breast-fed the baby right there, and he was sucking away like a madman an hour after his delivery. His Apgar score, a measure taken immediately after birth to assess a baby's initial health, was 9 out of 10.

McKenna put the bag with the cord blood into a box lined with bubble wrap to be picked up by a medical courier and shipped to Viacord, a storage facility in Kentucky, until the Trebings decided whether Katie would have a bone marrow transplant.

Steve was leery about the health of his newborn son. After what he and Stacy had gone through at Katie's birth, a relatively easy delivery seemed too good to be true. He wanted proof Christopher didn't have Diamond Blackfan anemia like his older sister. He wanted doctors to draw Christopher's blood and check it. Stacy talked him out of it.

"Prince Christopher," an elated Stacy said later of her new son. "Cal moves up to king."

Katie, now two and a half, and Calvin, now five, met their new brother in his hospital layette.

Katie seemed mystified. Stacy still had some stomach, and when Katie entered Stacy's hospital room and climbed onto her bed, she thought the baby was still inside her mom, even though she had just seen Christopher in the hall. "I want to see the baby," Katie said, pulling up Stacy's shirt.

"That's not the baby. That's Dunkin' Donuts and Mocha Frappuccino," Stacy said, laughing.

Calvin gave his mom a big hug; he'd brought her a stuffed dog that looked like Hobbes and a pink rose. Other members of Stacy and Steve's extended families arrived; nurses came in and said, "We want to see the miracle baby." To Stacy and Steve, that's exactly what Christopher seemed.

For the first few months after Christopher's birth, the Trebings focused on being a happy family of five. Stacy felt the instant bond she'd felt with Calvin and Katie; she melted when Christopher looked at her. Everything that had come before to orchestrate Christopher's birth, all the effort, all the medicine, all the science, all seemed moot. Steve still had the looming fear that something was going to be wrong with Christopher; he hoped every day that nothing would come up. After Katie's birth, everything had been so upside-down and shocking. "It instills the fear of God in you," Steve said.

But Christopher thrived. He got so big so fast that Steve and Stacy nicknamed him Bubba. He seemed to cry only when hungry, and even that was more whimper than demand. There were no nights spent pacing the hallways holding an inconsolable, wailing infant, as there had been with Calvin and Katie. There could be a circus going on and he'd sleep through it if he wanted, Stacy thought. Stacy later reported that she even fantasized about having a fourth child. By July, when Christopher was two months old, the Trebings were thoroughly enjoying the summer. Stacy had lost thirty-five pounds of her baby weight. Katie was doing well back on blood transfusions; she lost the weight she had gained while on steroids and shed her mood swings as well. Calvin and Katie went to summer day camp three days a week. That gave Stacy one-on-one time with Christopher.

Calvin and Katie were adjusting to a new member of the family. Calvin had an easier time than Katie. Katie didn't like it when Christopher got Stacy's attention.

"Put the baby down!" Katie demanded from time to time.

"So I can hold you?" Stacy asked once.

"Yeah," Katie said.

"Sit here," Stacy said, motioning next to her. "A little regression? You want to be the baby?"

"Yeah," Katie said, and she snuggled with Stacy on the couch.

"But babies can't go to camp," Stacy said.

Three months after Christopher's birth, Stacy and Steve took Katie to her regular appointment with Jeffrey Lipton, her Diamond Blackfan anemia doctor at Schneider Children's Hospital in New Hyde Park. By now, Katie had had more than thirty blood transfusions and couldn't go more than three weeks or so without one; she saw Lipton every six months for him to monitor her overall progress. At this visit, Lipton nudged the Trebings again to focus on Katie's treatment options. They needed to make a decision about a bone marrow transplant.

He reminded them that Katie's continuing blood transfusions were only a stopgap. A transplant was the best choice to give her the most normal life, he said.

It was time to act.

"If you ask me who is more likely to be alive in six months, the child with a transplant or a child with transfusions, the answer would be the child with transfusions," Lipton told them. "But," he added ominously, "if you ask me who will be alive in thirty years, the likelihood would be the child with the transplant." He mentioned a study that sobered the Trebings: only 57 percent of transfusion-dependent Diamond Blackfan patients were still alive at age forty. "If she were my granddaughter, I would encourage my son and his wife to do the transplant," Lipton told them.

Lipton gave the Trebings a tour of his hospital's transplant unit. Stacy couldn't get past the fact that she wouldn't be allowed to stay overnight with Katie there; Katie still wandered into bed with Stacy and Steve nearly every night. Stacy couldn't bear the thought of her daughter alone in the hospital overnight if she was really sick or suffering.

They went home depressed, and continued to lean against the option of a transplant. They were terrified Katie could die from transplant complications. Statistically, of every ten children who received bone marrow transplants from matched siblings, one child didn't survive. On top of that, Katie's pediatrician, Richard Ancona, was more conservative about a transplant.

"I would just leave her alone," Ancona told Stacy at one of Katie's checkups.

"Why?" Stacy asked.

"Because I think there is going to be something else that can help her in the future," Ancona said. Some new drug, some new treatment. Maybe even a cure.

Then there was Jack, the young son of Steve's childhood friend Pete McBride and his wife, Jen. Jack had leukemia and underwent a bone marrow transplant from a donor matched from the general population. Stacy and Steve learned firsthand how sick chemotherapy makes a child. Chemo is the first round of a transplant and in Katie's case would obliterate her Diamond Blackfan–tainted marrow. In the process, it would also wipe out her immune system, making her so weak the sniffles could kill her. The McBrides were a tremendous resource; they were close enough friends with the

Trebings that they had given them all the details, the good and the bad, and they told the Trebings what questions to be sure to ask doctors before settling on a transplant hospital for Katie. Stacy and Steve tried to tell themselves that Katie wouldn't have as hard a road as Jack did because Jack's body was already weak from the leukemia when he'd started the transplant. Despite his setbacks, Jack had made it through the transplant and was in his first year of recovery.

Steve and Stacy had been using the Camp Sunshine letter from Wendy Zangrando as a guide in their research. The letter could not be more blunt in warning parents about possible pitfalls in the transplant process. Steve had scrutinized every word in the letter, and his penciled notes marked up the margins. He brought it with him to Katie's doctor appointments. His notations reminded him to ask the doctors about getting Katie a liver biopsy to make sure her liver could withstand the transplant drug protocol, something the Zangrandos regretted they hadn't done with their son.

Steve made a note to research whether the transplant hospital had access to the experimental drug used to battle veno-occlusive disease, which had contributed to Keir Zangrando's death. Schneider Children's Hospital, where Lipton practiced, was not participating in that trial. That, to the Trebings, became an insurmountable negative.

The Trebings had to decide whether to jeopardize their daughter's life to save it. They went back and forth, back and forth. One day, they were sure they would do it. The next day, they wavered.

Lying awake at night, Stacy wondered, *How can I put Katie through this?* But, in her gut, it started to feel like the right thing. She knew she and Steve shouldn't drag out a decision—the more time passed, the more transfusions Katie would have and the more damaged her liver would be. What if they didn't do the bone marrow transplant, and Katie wound up needing a liver transplant? As Stacy reasoned, Katie was largely healthy now, her body strong and thus better able to tolerate the whole ordeal.

Steve wanted more information, something he could point to that would force him to decide this was transplant time. Even though it would be bad if Katie's iron counts climbed higher, Steve sometimes hoped that would happen, because that threat would make him feel he had no choice but to proceed. The temptation to avoid the transplant was enormous. But Steve's meticulous statistical research had shown him that Katie's best odds were in doing the transplant and doing it now. "Do it today to save tomorrow," he urged himself.

The Trebings' insurance provider gave them permission to explore four locations for Katie's possible transplant. The Trebings had already crossed Schneider Children's Hospital off their list, primarily due to the defibrotide issue. In October, the Trebings went to Children's Hospital Boston. They drove up in the morning and came back in the afternoon. The doctor they met with there agreed with Dr. Lipton: Katie's best bet was a transplant before the age of five.

On a blustery Veterans Day, Stacy and Steve drove into Manhattan to meet with Dr. Farid Boulad, associate attending pediatrician of the bone marow transplant service at Memorial Sloan-Kettering Cancer Center. Katie's disease was not cancer, but Sloan-Kettering also handled nonmalignant blood disorders. It was the third location the Trebings interviewed. They'd decide whether to visit the fourth—Cincinnati Children's Hospital Medical Center, where Keir Zangrando had his transplant—after today's meeting. Even though Keir hadn't survived his transplant, Cincinnati Children's Hospital Medical Center was still considered a top-notch hospital for transplants such as Katie's, and the Trebings wanted to see it for themselves.

20

"I Like This Place a Lot"

The pediatric waiting area at Sloan-Kettering evoked a theme park. Multicolored chairs were filled with children, many with surgical masks dotted with pictures of Donald Duck, many of them missing their hair. A tank filled with tropical fish had a statue of SpongeBob on the bottom. A waist-high wooden apple sat near the check-in counter painted in primary colors. A playroom was filled with toy trucks, games such as Chutes and Ladders, and tables for arts and crafts. The Trebings were called in for their consultation with Boulad, a bear of a man, although more teddy than grizzly. He had a dark beard with white whiskers in it and tortoiseshell glasses. A stethoscope was slung around his neck. Boulad launched into an overview of treatment options, which the Trebings had heard from Lipton and knew word for word. Boulad was blunt about what Katie would face during the six-week, in-hospital portion of the transplant regimen:

For the first ten days, Katie would have chemotherapy drugs to prepare her for transplant day, known widely as Day Zero. The chemo would cause disconcerting but short-term side effects, such as Katie's hair falling out. It could cause more permanent problems as well, such as infertility: the chemo could destroy her ovaries. It would also temporarily obliterate her immune system.

On Day Zero, Christopher's cord blood would be run through an intravenous line in Katie's chest. The transplant itself would be anticlimactic for Katie; she'd be awake and wouldn't feel anything. The doctors would do testing on Katie in advance to make a determination of whether Christopher's cord blood would be enough for a successful outcome. If Christopher's collected cord blood wasn't sufficient, doctors would have to use Christopher's bone marrow instead. In that case, he would come into the hospital on Day Zero. He would be put under general anesthesia, and bone marrow would be extracted from both his hips with a needle. Later the same day, the marrow itself, which looks like blood, would be dripped into Katie.

For fifteen days after the transplant day, Katie would be confined to her hospital room. Stacy and Steve could spend the day, and one parent could stay overnight, a huge relief to Stacy. Katie couldn't have any other visitors, and anyone who did enter her room, initially limited to Stacy, Steve, and hospital staff members, would have to don a gown, mask, and gloves. The parent staying overnight would sleep in them. At this stage, any infection could kill Katie.

Katie would get painful mouth sores, a side effect of the chemo drugs, and most likely would have to be fed intravenously because she would be too uncomfortable to eat. She might get fevers and need antibiotics. She might have diarrhea and nausea.

A host of threats could plague Katie up until she left the hospital:

Graft rejection. Katie's body might reject her brother's marrow, even though it was an exact match to hers.

Fatal infection.

Organ poisoning. The chemo drugs could be toxic to Katie's lungs, heart, liver, or kidneys, causing any or all to shut down.

Veno-occlusive disease, which shuts down the liver and contributed to the death of Keir Zangrando. Sloan-Kettering, however, did have access to defibrotide, the experimental drug to help fight veno-occlusive disease, Boulad told them. Steve and Stacy looked at each other with relief.

Katie could also develop complications such as acute graft-versus-host disease, in which Christopher's bone marrow attacked Katie's body, potentially setting off a number of complications including skin rashes, stomach problems, and liver issues. If severe, it could be fatal.

Hearing all this, Steve remained on the fence.

"He wants someone to say, 'You have to do it,'" Stacy said to Boulad.

"Nobody's going to say that," Boulad said. "I can tell you one other thing: if you go later, the transplant is more difficult than it is now." A catch-22. If parents waited for developments that convinced them a transplant was mandatory, those very developments made the transplant more dangerous.

Keeping Katie transfusion-dependent wasn't a perfect option either, Boulad reminded them. "Transfusion is far from being a hundred percent safe," he said. "We as physicians cannot make a decision for you. We can make a recommendation, and the recommendation is to go to transplant."

"When is the best time to do this?" Stacy asked.

"Between March and October," Boulad replied, adding that the hospital didn't do elective transplants in the winter because of a higher prevalence of respiratory viruses.

"What age would you recommend for her?" Stacy asked.

"Definitely less than five years of age. If you look at all the patients transplanted, regardless of disease, in patients less than five years old, the incidence of graft-versus-host disease is significantly less."

Another doctor saying younger than five, Steve thought.

But Boulad cautioned about transplanting a child who was too young. If the child's metabolism hadn't yet matured, the drugs were even more toxic.

"She's three," Stacy said. "So it could be this year or next year."

Boulad changed the subject to the issue of Christopher's cord blood.

Cord blood worked more effectively in leukemia patients than in children with diseases such as Diamond Blackfan, Boulad said. For Katie, cord blood presented a higher risk of graft rejection, he told them, something they hadn't heard before. Katie's T cells, the cells that fight foreign invaders, needed to be wiped out by chemo before a transplant, Boulad explained. In umbilical-cord blood, T cells are less mature. In theory, Katie's T cells, though severely depleted by chemo, might still be strong enough to overpower Christopher's cord T cells, causing rejection. So Boulad might want to use Christopher's bone marrow instead. He'd make that final call later.

"How old does Christopher have to be?" Stacy asked. "He's six months."

"The youngest donor I've collected marrow from was four months," Boulad said.

"Hopefully you wouldn't have to poke him so many times?" Stacy asked.

"The kids bounce back within twelve hours," Boulad said. "They're playing tag and running around. Adults walk around like this for two weeks." Boulad put his hands on the back of his hips as though they ached.

Once the transplant was complete, Katie's blood would have Christopher's DNA, Boulad said. "If she wants to get her brother in trouble, she could," he joked, meaning she could commit a crime and leave evidence making it appear it was Christopher who did it. Boulad laughed. "We've been watching too much *CSI*." Steve was once again awed by technology.

Boulad brought up one more point to consider. Like so many things before, this was jaw-dropping: he suggested having a doctor remove one of Katie's ovaries now to freeze it for possible future use.

The room went silent. They were talking about life—first Katie's, then her possible future child's. Cure one generation, preserve the next one.

Boulad explained doctors would remove one ovary by laparoscopy, through the belly button, at the same time they did Katie's pretransplant liver biopsy.

Stacy had seen a piece on ovary removal on the *Today* show one morning, but it had focused on older female cancer patients. She wondered now if Katie's eggs would be mature enough to be harvested.

"I will have to talk to Dr. Oktay to see if there's a minimum age," Boulad said.

"Would she be able to carry a child through a donor egg?" Stacy asked.

"Most probably yes," Boulad said. "It's happening more."

"Can I freeze my ovaries for her? I know there's a lot of ethical issues there...You don't think it's a good idea. I can see by the look on your face," Stacy said.

"I've never thought of that," Boulad said. "I need to think about it. Off the top of my head I don't see why not. But it would be a half-sibling for her."

"Kind of weird," Stacy said.

"A little bit," Boulad said. "It's the first time a person asked me that question. Mention it to Dr. Oktay as well."

Stacy looked at Steve. "You have any other questions?"

"No," Steve said.

"Your brain is full?" Stacy said.

"Getting there," Steve said.

"If we decide to start this process, what's the next step?" Stacy asked.

"Give me a call," Boulad said. He handed them a consent form they would have to sign if they went ahead. It was seven pages long.

When a date is set for transplant, he warned them, half the time there's something that postpones it. A runny nose, an infection.

On the way out, Boulad walked the Trebings around the pediatric unit. It had thirty-six rooms. Boulad had just run in the previous Sunday's New York City Marathon, in which 650 runners dedicated to Sloan-Kettering raised two million dollars. Steve knew all about the marathon; his tent company put up the tents at Manhattan's Tavern on the Green in Central Park, which was marathon central.

After the meeting, Steve and Stacy walked to the elevator, lost in thought. "We have to ultimately both end up at one hundred percent in favor of a transplant," Steve said.

"I don't know if I can get to one hundred percent," Stacy said. She was at 85 percent now.

"Me too," Steve said.

"I like this place a lot. I can sleep with her," Stacy said. "Part of me wants to just do it this March and get it done. Part of me wants to wait."

"What are you really waiting for?" Steve asked. "You're waiting for something else bad to happen?"

"If we do it now, she won't remember it as much," Stacy said. "The longer we wait, the more she'll remember it. Do you still want to go to Cincinnati? I don't think it's necessary." Sloan-Kettering felt like the right choice to Stacy.

"I don't either," Steve said. "Right now I feel very relieved."

But the temporary relief didn't make the Trebings' anxiety go away. Shortly after their meeting with Boulad, for instance, Steve and Stacy were on their way to a family gathering, and they had an enormous fight in the car about how little Stacy felt Steve was helping around the house. Stacy dropped Steve and the kids off and then drove around the block by herself for half an hour, trying to stop sobbing. Steve and Stacy didn't have time to talk about the argument afterward, but Stacy knew she didn't really care whether Steve helped fold the laundry—it was just the stress of all the decision making, and of what they knew awaited Katie and Christopher. Finding a place for the transplant was one big step. But it was only one step. The hardest was yet to come.

Over the next few weeks, there was no lightning-bolt moment when the Trebings decided, "We have to do this." The pendulum merely swung in the direction of going ahead with the transplant and then stayed there.

21

"Now It's Crunch Time"

Katie and her family and friends celebrated her third birthday in December of 2005 at the Palace in Smithtown, a storefront birthday center on the town's main street. The children frolicked on a moon bounce. Then they painted ceramic dolphins and ballet slippers and Batmobiles. Katie picked Ariel from *The Little Mermaid*. Calvin picked a three-headed monster. Piñatas and Mylar balloons hung everywhere. During a treasure hunt, Katie galloped around the room looking for clues, then walked the plank over a fake pond to choose candy prizes from a treasure chest. She chose a pink wristband that said DIVA. She played freeze dance and hula hoops. All the kids lined up and each said, "Happy birthday, Katie," into the microphone.

"This is a big birthday for us," Stacy had said before the party. It would be the year of Katie's bone marrow transplant. Katie made a wish in front of a candle on a cupcake decorated with pink fluffy frosting. She blew it out on the first try.

A few days after Katie's birthday, she was scheduled for her monthly blood transfusion at Stony Brook University Medical Center. Katie's number of transfusions was climbing up through the thirties now. When Stacy arrived with Katie, she got some startling news. Every time Katie was scheduled for a blood transfusion, she had to go to the hospital two days prior to have her blood typed and crossed with the donors' blood. This time when they did the testing, Katie's blood had shown antibodies to something called "little e," an antigen that 98 percent of the population, including her designated donors, had in their blood. That meant she could have a dangerous reaction if blood with this antigen was given to her; it meant that her body was starting to recognize that all this blood she was getting wasn't really hers.

Dr. Dennis Galanakis, director of blood services for Stony Brook, wanted to test Steve's and Christopher's blood to find out if their red blood cells had the little e, so Stacy called Steve. He drove over with the baby to meet them at the hospital. Sticking his arm out to get his blood drawn made Steve empathetic to what Katie had to go through every month. Christopher sat on Steve's lap when it was his turn, and he screamed through the procedure.

Stacy was confused, unsure of the implications of the news. Did this mean Katie couldn't get Christopher's bone marrow? Would there be enough blood donors without little e for Katie to still get blood transfusions? Galanakis assured Stacy that 2 percent of the population of the New York metropolitan area was still plenty of blood. "These kinds of problems happen in a blood bank like ours every day," he said. Stacy and Steve saw this as another sign pointing toward transplant and were relieved that Katie would need only a few more transfusions until she was done with them for life. Stacy was also relieved that Katie had an appointment scheduled in two weeks with Dr. Lipton; surely he would be able to explain the little-e issue to them in detail.

The nurses gave Katie a birthday cake; nurse Lori Seda dressed in an elf cap for Christmas. Stacy blew out the candles for Katie, and Katie watched *Polar Express* on a TV set as she ate her slice of cake and got her blood transfusion from the general population.

A few days after Christmas, a clown dressed as a physician— Dr. Schmendrick, to be exact—barged into the waiting room of Dr. Lipton's office at Schneider Children's Hospital. He wore a white lab coat, a round, red nose, and big floppy orange shoes. He and his female assistant—members of the Big Apple Circus Clown Care Unit, which wandered the hospital trying to make children laugh—put on a spontaneous fashion show. Katie and Steve watched from where they were sitting on the floor playing with a plastic kitchen set, waiting for Katie's appointment. Steve's sister, Nancy, was there as well; she had come with the Trebings to this appointment so she could entertain Katie if necessary.

"Don't disturb me while I'm trying to model," Dr. Schmendrick admonished the children. "I'm super modeling. You think it's easy walking down the runway and making millions of dollars?"

"Who made that outfit?" the girl assistant asked, setting him up for a joke.

"It's a Calvin Clown suit," Dr. Schmendrick said. "And a Vidal Buffoon hat."

The jokes didn't even make Stacy smile. She was too distracted, worried about a letter she'd received from her insurance company. Currently, the Trebings' health insurance company didn't have any hospital in its network that did pediatric bone marrow transplants, so the Trebings had their pick of places. But the letter informed the Trebings that as of January 1, 2006—three days from now—the health system that included Schneider Children's Hospital would be added to the plan. Stacy had an unsettling fear that the insurance company would give them a hard time about going to Sloan and tell them they had to go to Schneider instead.

A nurse popped into the waiting room. "Kathleen Trebing?" she said.

"Don't call her Kathleen," Stacy said. "She'll think you're either a teacher or a doctor. She goes by Katie."

"We'll note that in the chart," the nurse said.

Katie picked up the plastic food she'd been playing with and put it into a basket she could bring into the examining room with her. Dr. Lipton smiled as Katie entered with her basket. "I will have the T-bone and a nice cabernet if you've got that in there," he said. Steve, Nancy, and Stacy sat down, and Stacy jumped right in to asking about the issues facing Katie. "Can you explain to us what the little-e thing is? Did Dr. Galanakis tell you?"

"The blood bank did speak to me," Lipton said. Little e is a subcomponent in blood that 98 percent of people have, Lipton explained. "Katie doesn't have little e in her blood. When she got blood from someone who had little e, she made antibodies. In the future, she can't get little-e blood. Most people have little e. She finally got sensitized to it."

"What if Christopher has little e? How can he be Katie's bone marrow donor?" Stacy asked anxiously.

"If Chris has little e, you just have to take the red cells out of the product. A single antibody is not an issue. Blood-group incompatibilities aren't a cause for rejection," Lipton reassured her and Steve. "It just makes the transfusion type and cross match a little more difficult."

"So ninety-eight percent of the population has little e," Steve said. "So she's down to two percent."

"Our directed donors are out," Stacy said. "We're back to the general pool?"

"I always said the general pool was fine," Lipton said.

Stacy then broke the news to Dr. Lipton that she and Steve were going to take Katie to Sloan-Kettering rather than Schneider's transplant unit. She felt like Lipton was her dad, and she didn't want to upset him with their choice. "Are you okay with that?" she asked.

"I'd rather do it here," Lipton said.

"We want to do it with you guys, but we really don't like the transplant unit. I can't stay with Katie," Stacy said.

"I want you to be comfortable," Lipton said. "The most important thing is this isn't a hundred percent guaranteed success. The cure rate is ninety-two point five percent. In school, ninety-two point five percent is good. As a parent...you've got to be one hundred percent comfortable with your choice." Lipton explained to Stacy that if the transplant wasn't successful, he wouldn't want her to resent his hospital because she had been deprived of sleeping with her daughter during her final days. "We want you to be comfortable with the decision. That is the most important thing."

Katie was sitting on her aunt Nancy's lap putting bug stickers on pages. Lipton turned his attention to Katie. "Can I feel your belly?" he asked.

"No," Katie said.

"I'm just going to touch your belly," Lipton said, as Stacy led her daughter to the examining table. Lipton had to feel Katie's liver to see whether it was becoming enlarged. Katie cried and flailed. "No boo-boo. No boo-boo," Stacy whispered in Katie's ear, reassuring her that she wasn't going to be poked with any needles. Lipton pronounced Katie's liver fine.

"That's just touching her belly," Steve said of Katie's reaction. "Imagine when the other stuff comes."

Stacy asked Lipton's opinion of the possibility of removing one of Katie's ovaries.

Lipton was skeptical. "There's very little data on girls under ten and whether the eggs could be used to accomplish a pregnancy when she is in her twenties and thirties. If it doesn't work the way they're expecting it to work, you've taken away half her eggs."

Steve said he'd thought that after the chemotherapy, none of the eggs would be usable and she'd be sterile.

"She's going to definitely have fewer eggs. She's definitely at risk of infertility," Lipton said. "But the ovary does two things: eggs and hormones. What's the impact of taking an ovary from a child? I suspect the answer is going to be 'We don't know.'" Nobody had studied how the loss of one ovary might complicate her sexual development in terms of the ability to produce hormones and the possibility of very early menopause.

"We're thinking March we're hopefully starting this whole procedure. Do you want to see her again before that?" Stacy asked.

"Just keep in touch," Lipton said. "You're in good hands; I don't think there's any need to see her before then."

The Trebings left the hospital. It was raining, and water stains seeped down the huge, concrete hospital building like icing over the sides of a cake. Drops crept down the blue, orange, and yellow Keith Haring sculpture in the front courtyard. The flag was plastered to the flagpole.

The Trebings spent Christmas Eve with their families. Stacy and Steve traditionally hosted; Stacy's father would sneak out at a certain point, change into a Santa suit, and come back to the house to leave a sack of presents on the lawn as the children watched from the living room windows. On Christmas Day, Katie and Calvin both got hermit crabs; Bubba got clothes and was more interested in the wrapping paper.

New Year's Eve the Trebings spent alone with their children. Steve fell asleep at ten. As the clock neared midnight, Stacy sat at her computer alone to send out a New Year's e-mail to family and friends. Together Steve and Stacy had come to a decision, a decision to move forward and schedule the transplant. They had told their friends and family members. Now it was time to prepare for what was to come.

Happy New Year to all, she wrote, tears streaming down her face.

As you know, I tend to downplay most things and have really not been focusing on the upcoming months, as I wanted to enjoy the holidays. Well, the holidays are over and now it's crunch time.

I am anxious to speak to a psychologist. I do not know how to explain to Cal what Katie will be going through and why Mom and Dad will be gone. I am tormented with how to explain to Katie that she cannot go home and see her brothers, or why she will be going through this process.

So if you talk to us and ask us, "How's Katie? How's everything?" we will probably say good. And the day to day is, but internally it's really not, but we may not want to talk about it and sometimes maybe we do.

As it is almost midnight and 2006, I can honestly say, as much as I don't want my kids to get older, I can't wait for 2007 and to look behind and say "Thank you God for watching over my family and helping us get through this difficult time." And most of all for Katie to say, "Happy New Year, Mommy." Wishes to all for a healthy New Year. Love, Stacy.

22

"You Conceived Your Son for This?"

The Trebings' last piece of research was to meet with Dr. Kutluk Oktay, the doctor at New York–Presbyterian Hospital/Weill Cornell Medical Center who would be the one to freeze Katie's ovary if the Trebings decided to have it surgically removed. He listened as Steve and Stacy explained Katie's upcoming bone marrow transplant.

"We have the cord blood of my son, who is eight months old, who is an exact HLA match," Stacy said.

"You conceived your son for this?" Oktay asked candidly.

"Well, we wanted...," Stacy began.

"You wanted another baby, so why not?" Oktay finished. "So you're going to use cord blood for it?"

"They may have to take some of his marrow, but mostly the cord," Stacy said. She was still hoping that Boulad would go with the cord blood and that Christopher wouldn't be physically involved at all.

Then Oktay changed the subject to Katie's future fertility. "As far as transplant, your child will be getting large doses of chemotherapy, drugs that are known to have a negative impact on ovarian function. It would be close to impossible to think she would get to an age to have her own babies before getting ovarian failure."

"She has the RPS nineteen gene for DBA. Fifty percent of her children will also be affected by the disease," Stacy said.

"In the long run, she may be another PGD candidate," Oktay said. Doctors would use the same procedure they used to select Christopher to select an embryo of Katie's that didn't have DBA. "That's a very good reason to do PGD."

Oktay went on to explain how the ovary would be removed, cut into strips with the eggs still embedded inside, and frozen. How females are born with all the eggs they will ever have, and they lose them with age. In a three-year-old, one ovary probably has five hundred thousand eggs, Oktay explained. Even if in the freezing process Katie lost half of those, that still left two hundred and fifty thousand eggs, equivalent to the fertility level of a normal twenty-five-year-old, Oktay said.

In the future, when Katie was ready to have children, doctors would either replace the ovary in its normal location or surgically implant it under the skin in her forearm or abdomen. They would give Katie the same hormones and other drugs that women took to stimulate their ovaries during the in vitro fertilization process, and then extract eggs and fertilize them in the laboratory.

The procedure was experimental. No woman who'd had her ovary taken out at age three had yet returned to have it reimplanted. In fact, doctors had reimplanted cryopreserved ovaries in very few women worldwide; three of them had given birth, Oktay told the Trebings. Other extracted ovaries were still frozen until the women were ready for them.

"The freezing part is pretty much standard and established now. The research is how to put it back in," Oktay said. "A lot of countries have been doing this only the past three to four years and the patients are not ready to take the ovaries back yet.

"This gives you hope," Oktay said. "It may not result in any benefit to her because it's so new. We may find out in ten years it's not efficient, and we're not doing it anymore. But the other side is about guaranteed zero." The main risk, Oktay told them, was the risk associated with any surgery. But Katie was already going through surgery to have her liver biopsied, so adding the ovary removal during the same surgical procedure wouldn't add any significant danger, he said.

Stacy wanted to know about other possible ways that Katie could have a child at least partially linked to her biologically. "What about me? Could I go through another IVF cycle and you could take my eggs and freeze them for her? I've already done two cycles, why not another one?"

"That's an interesting option. We've never done that. That is potentially possible," Oktay said. "Obviously there has to be some discussion about that. Grandma at the same time is mother…always there are these social and ethical questions about this." Oktay went out on a limb, joking, "You could have another child through IVF/PGD that's a girl, and she could be the egg donor in the future."

"Dr. Stelling won't do that," Stacy quickly said. "He won't select a boy or girl."

Steve asked whether putting the ovary back in a different place could increase Katie's odds for ovarian cancer. "We don't know," Oktay said. "There are not enough cases. When you decide to do this, you're signing a research consent form."

The decision to remove one of Katie's ovaries was far easier than the decision to go to transplant. Katie was having liver surgery anyway; they might as well have her ovary preserved. The Trebings could worry about whether to put it back in when Katie was older. By then, there would be twenty more years of research.

"It seems like a win-win situation," Steve said.

"It seems like you're using every piece of recent technology to your benefit," Oktay said.

"Poor kid," Stacy said about Katie.

"Poor kid, but lucky kid," Oktay amended. "Ten years ago you could do none of this. Cord blood. PGD. Ovarian preservation."

On the way home in the car, the Trebings talked about the cost—they had to put down five thousand dollars out of pocket because the ovarian surgery was considered experimental and wasn't covered by insurance. Their families and friends had been asking to do a fund-raiser to help Steve and Stacy with all of Katie's medical expenses. But the Trebings were better off financially than many of their friends. They had just taken a vacation to Grand Bahama; they felt uncomfortable asking for help. And yet the medical costs would soon wipe out their savings. They'd already spent more than thirty-five thousand dollars to have Christopher.

They decided to let their families run a fund-raiser. Stacy called her friend Michelle Weinkauf. Stacy and Michelle had attended physical therapy school together. Michelle had been asking to spearhead a fund-raiser with Stacy's sisters, and Stacy left her a voice message giving her consent.

Meanwhile, Steve and Stacy had some last loose ends to tie up to feel 100 percent good about their decision to go to transplant. Steve was still looking at statistics and calculations; Stacy was searching her gut. She called Dr. Blanche Alter at the National Cancer Institute. Alter was another expert on DBA; the Trebings had met her at Camp Sunshine. She said the only thing she would do differently was try steroids one more time. Most likely Katie wouldn't respond because she didn't last time, but there was a chance she might. Then the Trebings would have to decide if they were willing to live with the long-term side effects of steroids, which included osteoporosis, cataracts, diabetes, and weight gain. If it didn't work the second time, then she would do the transplant.

Despite their occasional stresses and fights, Stacy and Steve felt their research bringing them closer in their marriage. They stayed up many nights talking about it. It wasn't something they could avoid; they had to focus together and work as a team. They discussed Dr. Alter's advice to try steroids a second time, but they agreed that even if it worked, they would rather Katie not have to live with the side effects of the steroids that seemed to turn her into a different girl. That meant they were ready to go to transplant right away.

One night, as Stacy was putting Katie to sleep, she decided it was time to start breaking the news to Katie about the transplant.

"Do you want to not have to do your boo-boo anymore?" Stacy asked Katie, referring to the blood transfusions.

"Yes," Katie said. "No more boo-boo."

It broke Steve's heart that Katie was so eager to get rid of the boo-boos. It wasn't even the monthly transfusions—she was up to a total of forty now—that were the worst. It was the nightly Desferal injections. Stacy and Steve did everything they could to make them less painful—thirty minutes before the injection, for instance, they smeared EMLA cream in a big circle on Katie's thigh to numb the skin. Then they waited until Katie was asleep to inject her, to avoid her high anxiety. About 50 percent of the nights, things went well. But half the time, Katie woke up screaming and crying. And the process caused her painful leg cramps. And then there was the morning—Katie hated taking the needle out as much if not more than putting it in.

"We have to go to the hospital for a couple of days then," Stacy said.

Katie rolled over and started whimpering. "Mommy, I don't want to go to the hospital," Katie said. Stacy dropped the subject, deciding that right before bed wasn't the best time for heavy conversations with her three-year-old.

A few nights later, when Steve was putting the Desferal pump needle into Katie's thigh, it was hard to get the needle inserted correctly and Katie was really in pain. As she was crying, Steve asked her if she wanted to stop getting the nightly needles. "All you have to do is go to the hospital with Daddy and Mommy and we'll fix it," Steve assured her.

"Can we go now?" Katie asked. Steve felt incredible relief. As much as Katie hated going to the hospital, she would've gone that night if it meant no more Desferal needles. Katie was on board for the bone marrow transplant.

––––––––––

The first fund-raiser meeting was at the end of January, across the street from Stacy's house at her sister Lisa's. A dozen of Stacy and Steve's friends and family members gathered at Lisa's dining room table.

"This is really, really, really awkward for us," Stacy said. She started to cry. "The whole thing is really weird. We want to let everyone know Steve and I were first against this because we have a lovely home and a wonderful family. As things are going by, the money is going. Everyone's been asking about this...The whole thing is very strange for our family to be asking for outside help."

"It's about time," Michelle interrupted.

"You two are two of the most giving, loving people we've ever met," piped in Adrienne Law, who had been one of Stacy's high-school classmates.

"You would be the first people to step up to the plate to help us," Michelle said.

Pete McBride had been one of two best men at Stacy and Steve's wedding. He knew what they were feeling because of Jack's bone marrow transplant the previous year, which he was still recovering from. Their family had a fund-raiser a year ago and went through the same soul-searching, wondering if it was okay to have a fund-raiser if they weren't poor.

"People get ruined even with good insurance," he said. "The fund-raiser isn't for you." It's for Katie, he said. People come because a child needs help. If they don't think you should be having a fund-raiser, they won't come. And Katie would need health support even in the future, after the transplant, he pointed out. The chemotherapy affects teeth, for instance, and she might need extensive dental work in the future, he said. About six hundred people had come to Jack's fund-raiser, and he said the Trebings should expect the same.

They got down to business, planning where the fund-raiser

could be. The firehouse, someone threw out. The Moose Lodge. The Smithtown Sheraton. People volunteered to call each place. They tossed around ideas of admission prices and raffles.

"My uncle owns a B and B in Ireland. We can raffle off a trip to Ireland," Jane Ann McBride said.

"That's an awesome gift," said Jeff McNamara, who had been Steve's other best man and who played with him on his darts team.

Fifty dollars was suggested as a ticket price. Stacy's sister Leslie Giordanella looked skeptical. "It's not a lot," Michelle said.

"Some people buy the ticket and don't even come," Jeff said. "What's the time frame on this?"

"Unfortunately we're still waiting on insurance approval," Stacy explained. "We're supposed to be scheduled for the beginning of March."

"So it's tight. We've got to get things going," Jeff said.

After the business was completed, everyone ate chocolate chip cookies Lisa had baked. Pete and Steve talked about the amazing overlaps in their families. Pete's sister Jane Ann had brought Stacy and Steve together. Jack had been born on the exact same day as Calvin. Pete remembered parking his car next to the Trebings' car in the hospital emergency room parking lot. Now Jack and Katie both needed bone marrow transplants.

Stacy left to give Katie her Desferal needle. The next morning, Stacy would take Katie to Stony Brook University Medical Center for transfusion no. 41. Over the weekend, Stacy planned to take Katie for a haircut, the first of two she would get before her transplant. Stacy wanted to gradually transition Katie from her long hair to a short bob, so that when her hair fell out during the transplant process it wouldn't be as shocking or as messy.

On Monday, February 6, Stacy got a letter from her insurance company. She unfolded the sheet of paper; it was the news she'd been fearing. The company approved Katie's transplant, but not the hospital. Memorial Sloan-Kettering? Denied. Katie should go to Schneider Children's Hospital on Long Island instead, now an in-network facility.

The letter made Stacy sob. She felt misled. The insurance company had allowed them to research other facilities and then took away the option of having the transplant at one of them. The decision to go to transplant was not an easy one, but Stacy and Steve had finally come to terms with moving forward. Memorial Sloan-Kettering was the only hospital they felt completely comfortable with, and now that was in jeopardy of being eliminated. If the Trebings disagreed with the decision, they had to file an appeal. "It's not about comfort. It's not about preference. It's all about medical necessity," Stacy explained to Steve when she called him at work and broke the news to him. "We have to make the case that Memorial Sloan-Kettering is medically necessary."

Steve was livid. "Where are these people?" he asked Stacy. "I think they're on Long Island. I'm going there, and I'm going to take my daughter." He wanted to hand-deliver the appeal.

Stacy calmed Steve down, at least temporarily. The way she saw it, there were two compelling medical reasons to go to Sloan. Number one, Sloan-Kettering had access to defibrotide while Schneider didn't. And number two, Dr. Oktay could do the ovary removal.

While Steve was still at work, Stacy got on the phone. First, she called Dr. Lipton at Schneider. He agreed with their decision to go to Memorial Sloan-Kettering, but he couldn't officially, in writing, side with her—in effect, he would be stating that his facility couldn't do a DBA bone marrow transplant when they'd already successfully done many. He was in an awkward position, Stacy realized. Still, she was sick to her stomach. She wanted a hospital that had access to the experimental drug defibrotide, and there were only a handful of those. *I'm not compromising for Katie,* Stacy thought. *There's no room for error here.*

Stacy started making a list of other reasons the insurance company should let them go to Sloan instead of making them go to Schneider. Sloan-Kettering had world-renowned, long-term follow-up care. Sloan had done 4,000 bone marrow transplants. Schneider, a much newer institution, had only done 120.

When Steve got home, the Trebings put the three kids to bed upstairs and came back down to talk strategy. They headed to the basement and started printing out information from the Internet. They'd get letters from Katie's pediatrician, her hematologist at Stony Brook. From Dr. Oktay. They'd ask to have the letters faxed to them to put their appeal packet together as quickly as possible.

"Is someone crying up there?" Steve asked suddenly.

It was Christopher. They stopped everything to listen for a minute, and he settled down.

"The first thing I want to ask them is 'Do you have kids?'" Steve said. "And depending on their response to us, I'll have people ready to picket outside their office. That will fire them up."

"You and your picketing," Stacy teased. To her, it seemed Steve had morphed into Erin Brockovich. "You better put some padding in your bra, honey," she ribbed.

Steve took a break to lift weights on a weight bench. "I'm going to knock them out in the first round," he said. He looked over at Stacy, who had been up since early that morning when the kids awoke. "You look like shit," he joked.

But that was exactly how she felt.

23

"Will I Get Handcuffed with My Kids?"

"Can you hold on?" the insurance company representative said again.

Stacy had been trying in vain to get a supervisor from the insurance company to talk to her on the phone. She called first thing in the morning, and every time she would ask the customer service clerk a question, she'd be put on hold while the clerk tried to get an answer. But when she asked for a supervisor, she was told none was available. *She's putting me on hold to find out what she needs to know,* Stacy thought. *So who is she finding out* from*? Her supervisor.*

Stacy just wanted to know if the review would take forty-eight hours or forty-five days—whether they'd get an answer in time to go ahead with Katie's transplant this year. The clerk came back on the line. "Because this is a grievance case, we will review it within forty-eight hours," she said.

Stacy felt like the clouds had finally parted and the light was shining through. At least she and Steve would get an answer to their appeal quickly. She looked at Christopher, and he gurgled at her. *Thank God he's such a good baby, giving me his little smile while these ladies are killing me,* Stacy thought.

By Wednesday afternoon Stacy and Steve had collected all but one of the letters they needed. They were just waiting on the one from the hematologist at Stony Brook who had replaced Dr. Mueller when Mueller moved to Los Angeles.

In the midst of the chaotic week, Stacy and Katie carried out a volunteer commitment they'd made for Katie to appear in Stony Book University Hospital's poster campaign encouraging people to give blood. They headed up to the roof of the hospital for the photo shoot with the Stony Brook girls' softball team and the Stony Brook mascot, a wolf; a college student wore the wolf costume, complete with a furry head and red eyes. Katie held a baseball and glove as the softball team members gathered around her. "You're with the whole softball team! Wait until Daddy finds out. Say cheese," Stacy said.

"I don't like the wolf," Katie said. The student took his hand out of the wolf glove and showed Katie that it was a human hand, but that didn't help. "We don't have to go near him," Stacy said to Katie. "We'll stay here."

"Katie, right here, look at the camera, Katie," the photographer said.

"She's so cute," said the coordinator of marketing promotion for Stony Brook's athletic department. "Do you think she'd like it if they signed a ball for her? Not today, but we'll get it for her."

"Would you like that, Katie? If all these girls signed a ball for you? You could keep it in your room," Stacy said. Katie nodded. They finished the photo shoot at two forty-five that afternoon. Stacy went home hoping that the final letter would be waiting for her. But it hadn't arrived yet.

On Friday morning at ten thirty on February 10, four days after they had received the insurance company's rejection letter saying they couldn't go to Sloan-Kettering, Stacy and Steve were ready to hand in their appeal. The company indeed had an office within driving distance, so Stacy got in the minivan with Katie and Christopher and headed there while Steve went to work. Katie walked in beside Stacy, who was pushing Christopher in his stroller; they were accompanied by the local newspaper reporter and photographer who had been covering Katie's story for more than eighteen months and who frequently went with the Trebings to medical and other appointments to document their quest. Stacy passed through the glass doors of the lobby and handed her paperwork to the receptionist who sat behind the counter.

Just then, an employee walked into the conference room adjacent to the lobby, and a group of her coworkers yelled, "Surprise!"

"It's a party," Stacy said to the receptionist. "Can we go?"

"One of the employees is getting married," the receptionist explained.

"I'd like to ask a question," Stacy said. "Can you get me someone who can answer it?"

The receptionist made a phone call and then hung up. "No one is available in customer service," she said.

Stacy glanced to the conference room packed with employees. "They're back there," Stacy said. "Should I get on my cell phone and call them? I don't want to give you a hard time. I just need to speak to someone. Anyone."

The receptionist said she couldn't help any further but could only take the appeal and hand it later to the right person.

"This is ludicrous," Stacy said, and she dialed the customer service phone number from her cell phone and asked for one of the employees she'd dealt with during the week. She was put on hold. Katie was eating Cheerios, and by this time, Christopher, who was now in Stacy's arms as she balanced her cell phone, was squirming.

"I can take the paperwork for you and they will call you," the receptionist said again.

A woman walked out of the conference room where the party was taking place.

"Are you in customer service?" Stacy asked her.

"No, I'm sorry, I'm not. I work in the marketing department," the woman said and disappeared through another door.

The receptionist interrupted.

"Mrs. Trebing, I really don't want to be rude, but I have your papers. I need to ask you to leave the reception area. I will give your papers to the appeals department. I need for you to leave the reception area, please."

Stacy put Christopher on the floor. She was still on her cell phone. "I'm on hold right now. They said they're going to get her," she said.

The receptionist made her own phone call. "I have a member in the lobby," she said. "I've taken the appeals papers and asked them to leave the area and they're not responding."

Christopher was crawling across the floor. Stacy was still on hold.

"Will I get handcuffed with my kids?" Stacy asked the receptionist. "I don't want to get you in trouble. I'll wait out in the hallway if that makes it better for you. I'm not here to get anybody in trouble. I'm just here to make my case."

A man walked out of the back office and into the lobby. He eyed the local reporter and photographer who had arrived with Stacy. "I'm working as a consultant here," he said to Stacy. "Can we talk inside?"

"Can you tell me your name?" Stacy said. "I just want to know who I'm talking to."

"Can you come inside and we can talk?"

A security guard appeared in the lobby. The reporter and photographer were escorted outside the glass double doors of the lobby. Tension was high as the consultant brought Stacy inside, into a small room with a couple of chairs. He sat her down and left the room, and she could hear him outside the door talking, telling two employees before they came into the room with him to stick to going over policy and procedures.

The employees didn't introduce themselves to Stacy as they entered. They wouldn't give her their full names when Stacy asked.

"Let me tell you what the procedure is," the consultant said, trying to establish the upper hand.

Stacy went back and forth with the employees for almost half an hour. Finally she got them to at least tell her when she might hear back—whether the forty-eight hours meant two days or two *business* days. She'd hear by Tuesday, they said.

When all this is over, Stacy thought, *I'm going to call back the com-*

pany and tell them how badly they handled this. She couldn't believe they'd escalated it into an antagonistic situation. *They just sent a pit bull out at me. They should've sent the pussycats,* she thought. It was a good thing Steve hadn't come with her because he would have been livid at how she was treated and would already be organizing the picketers, Stacy thought.

Stacy went home but didn't feel any relief. If the company turned her down, she and Steve would switch their insurance to a group that allowed her to go to Sloan-Kettering. But they would have to wait until the January 1 enrollment period to do that, and that meant Katie couldn't have the transplant until the following spring. Mentally, Stacy wasn't prepared to wait a whole extra year. And she didn't want Katie to.

Steve was relieved that at least he didn't have to stay up until two in the morning anymore pulling together their appeal. He hadn't done any work in two days. The only silver lining was that doing all the research had eliminated any doubts that he might have had that Memorial Sloan-Kettering was the right place for Katie.

Stacy tried to control her frustration that she'd spent the past week stressed out and working on the appeal instead of spending quality time with the three kids in the short time they had before Katie was scheduled to go into the hospital to start the process. *If something ever happens to Katie and this is the time I spent beforehand, I'll be really angry,* Stacy thought. But then she remembered her mantra, her promise, her prayer and said it aloud: "Everything will be fine."

On Monday afternoon, Stacy got a phone call from one of the women who had been in the room at the insurance company with her on Friday morning. "I have a decision," she said.

"What is it?" Stacy asked.

"I have to fax it to you," she said.

Stacy used her cell phone to call Steve and told him to stand by the fax machine in his office.

"It's not going through," the woman told Stacy.

Steve, standing by the fax machine, saw the words *fax failed*. Four times.

Unable to stand the suspense, Stacy went upstairs to retrieve a fax machine from under her bed that she'd been meaning to get rid of for two years. She plugged it in, and it worked. She watched as the decision printed out. Stacy grabbed the fax as it slid out of the machine and skimmed it—Katie had been approved for the pretransplant workup at Memorial Sloan-Kettering.

24

"This Is Mind-Boggling"

Stacy wasn't entirely sure what it meant to be approved for the workup. Would Katie then be allowed to go for transplant as well? Or would there be another round of decision making by the insurance company?

But it was a good sign, Stacy decided. She immediately picked up the phone, called Sloan-Kettering, and made an appointment for as soon as possible—three days from then: Thursday, February 16, 2006. This time, it wouldn't be just Stacy and Steve on a fact-finding mission. Katie and Christopher would be with them for initial examinations.

On Thursday morning, Stacy met first with Sean Jones, who was in charge of the insurance paperwork at Sloan-Kettering. Christopher sat on her lap. Steve went to the playroom with Katie, hoping to get her to fall in love with what they'd been calling "the big hospital." Katie was issued a surgical mask with Mickey Mouse on it, a precaution used to protect the immunocompromised children there from any viruses she might be carrying. Katie headed for the play stove area.

"This little gentleman's name is?" Jones said.

"Christopher," Stacy replied.

"Birthday?" Jones said.

"May fourth, 2005."

"What are the big plans for the birthday this year?" Jones asked.

"Probably nothing. Katie will probably still be recovering. He had a big christening."

"Next year," Jones said.

Stacy could tell Jones was used to speaking to distraught parents of children with life-threatening diseases; he was thorough yet soft-spoken and empathetic. When Jones was finished with Stacy, the four Trebings were called into Dr. Boulad's office.

"This must be Kathleen," Dr. Boulad said.

"We call her Katie," Stacy said.

"Give me five," Boulad said, and Katie did. She smiled.

"We did it," Stacy said, alluding to the insurance victory.

"So far," Dr. Boulad said.

"So far," Stacy repeated. "It's just pretransplant. We don't have approval for transplant yet. Do they usually do that? Break it up like that?"

"No. Sean is very optimistic. There should not be an issue," Boulad said.

They set Katie's liver biopsy and ovary removal for February 22, only a week away. Katie would be hospitalized overnight. One piece of tissue would go to a lab at the Mayo Clinic. They would look for how much iron was in a gram of dry tissue. The tissue would also be tested to see how scarred the liver already was. Katie would get a rank of 1 to 4 in each category, the lower, the better. If the numbers came back 3s or 4s, then the chemotherapy protocol would change a little bit. They would have to add an additional drug that might be more toxic to Katie in some ways but that would protect her liver. Both results should be back within a week of the surgery, Boulad told Stacy and Steve.

Christopher threw a toy mirror he'd been playing with onto the floor. Dr. Boulad picked it up. Christopher smiled and reached for it. "I know you want attention," Boulad said to Christopher. "I know. I've had my own. I've been there."

The major goal of today's testing of Katie and Christopher would be to confirm that Christopher was indeed an exact HLA match for Katie. "What you need to hear from me is that it's a ten-out-of-ten match," Boulad said. Katie and Christopher would each have blood drawn. Boulad jokingly covered his mouth to blur the words *blood count* so Katie wouldn't catch on that she would soon be stuck with a needle.

"It's not twelve out of twelve?" Stacy asked. She knew from her research that there were twelve HLA antigens.

"America is ten out of ten. Europe does twelve out of twelve. The two that are added in Europe are not important," Boulad said.

Katie was lying across Steve's lap now and Steve was tickling her tummy. Then Katie wanted to kiss Christopher.

"Aw," said Boulad.

"That can change at any time," Stacy warned.

"Been there too," Boulad said.

Steve shifted gears. "Just so I can let my parents know this...they'll be moving into my house," Steve said. "After the twenty-second, is there some kind of expectation of when we might be going in for chemo?"

"The week of the sixth of March probably, if all goes well. If there are any delays, then the following week." Katie would come into Sloan-Kettering prior to beginning chemotherapy to have a central line put into her chest. The line would be inserted into a large vein in Katie's chest so that medicine could be run directly into her bloodstream and also so that doctors could easily withdraw the blood they needed every day to monitor Katie's progress. In addition to more effectively delivering the medications, the central line saved the child the pain of constantly being poked with needles.

"If all goes well and everything goes smoothly," Boulad began.

Stacy interrupted. "*When* everything goes well and everything goes smoothly," she corrected.

Boulad began again. "*When* everything goes well and everything goes smoothly, we can take it out."

Dr. Rachel Kobos, a hematology/oncology fellow working under Boulad, started doing a routine exam on Christopher.

"Isn't he just the happiest boy?" Kobos said.

"Yes, he's the best," Stacy agreed.

Boulad kissed Christopher's toes. Christopher was laughing. He touched Boulad's face.

"Don't you dare pull this beard. You'll be in deep trouble," Boulad said.

Boulad instructed Stacy to put EMLA cream onto both Katie's and Christopher's arms in anticipation of the blood drawing. Katie knew what the cream meant.

"I want to go home," she said.

"This is going to be your home," Steve said to Katie.

"No, it's not," Katie said.

"For a little while," Steve said. "Mommy and Daddy will be here too."

"We'll decorate your room," Stacy added. "There'll be a TV in it. You can watch *Ice Age* whenever you want." That was one of Katie's favorite movies.

Katie began whimpering on Steve's lap. "I don't want to," she said.

"We're going to let them take a little blood and then we'll get ice cream and then go home. Should Christopher go first or you go first?" Stacy asked Katie, alluding to the blood tests.

"Christopher," Katie said.

"You don't want to show him how good you do it?" Stacy asked.

"No," Katie said. "Christopher first."

"You are ferocious," Dr. Boulad said.

"You haven't seen anything yet," Steve warned.

It was a long procedure taking Christopher's blood; it took the nurses more than forty-five minutes to find a viable vein and draw the seven tubes of blood that were needed. Steve started out holding Christopher on his lap in the phlebotomy room. Christopher watched *SpongeBob* on the television set as a nurse, Carlene Edwards, pushed on the veins of his right arm, trying to decide which would be best to take blood from.

She called over another nurse, Danielle Gehshan, to help hold Christopher still.

Christopher was crying, and his face was red. He was afraid, not in pain. He flailed his head back and forth. "He knows something is up," Steve said. Christopher tried to pull Gehshan's hand off him.

Stacy popped in. "Do you want me to do it with him?" She'd gone through this so many times with Katie, she had some comforting tricks up her sleeve.

"Sure," Steve said, handing Christopher over to Stacy and leaving with Katie.

Stacy gave Christopher a bottle, and he took it. Stacy sang the theme from *SpongeBob* to Christopher softly.

"They're chubby," Carlene Edwards said apologetically to Stacy. "Their veins are usually deeper, and smaller. They roll a lot, they move a lot. It's getting them in an ideal position and finding a vein." Stacy already knew all about that. Stacy told the nurses— there were four working on Christopher now—that when Katie first started blood transfusions, it often took the nurses seven sticks to find a vein. "They had to put a warm pack on to bring more fluid to the veins and make them fatter," she said.

"You're being so brave. So brave," Stacy said to Christopher.

Edwards looked at Christopher's right foot near his ankle; she put alcohol on there. "All right, we're going to probe him," she warned Stacy.

Blood started to flow out.

"We got it, Bubba. We got it," Stacy said.

Stacy had her head on Christopher's chest. He was screaming and squirming.

They finished filling the last tube, and Christopher fell asleep in Stacy's arms.

"You guys were in there awhile," Steve said when Stacy and Christopher emerged.

"They couldn't find a vein," Stacy said. This would remain a big problem for Christopher. But the results later confirmed Christopher was indeed a perfect ten-out-of-ten match for Katie.

That night, the fund-raising team met at Lisa's house. Jeff McNamara and his girlfriend helped Steve's dad put together a rocking horse that someone had donated for the raffle. Lisa's den was packed with other donations: a surfboard, a painting of a bull, a remote-control car, a Scrabble game, a basket of CDs. A dartboard donated from Steve's dart league.

Stacy came in. "Oh my gosh. Wow," she said when she saw the packed den. She told Jeff and Steve's dad how Katie had thrown up all over the car on the way home from Sloan-Kettering, and about the ordeal taking blood from Christopher's vein.

"I thought Christopher was done now, no?" Jeff said.

"Well, they have to make sure he's a match," Stacy said.

Jen McBride, Pete's wife, was there working. Their son, Jack, had stayed home. Easter Day would mark one year post-transplant, and he still had to stay away from crowds of people. She asked Stacy how Katie liked Sloan-Kettering.

"She was good today. She likes her new doctors. She likes the playground. It's like camp," Stacy said.

"Camp Sloan," Jen said.

"She's going in Tuesday for an ovary removal. This is all new, all experimental. They're going to take one of her ovaries. She's going to be sterile because of the chemo."

Stacy's friend Jill Kaplan was listening; her jaw dropped. "My God, this never ends. This is just mind-boggling," she said.

"Ovary freezing is really, really new," Stacy said. "I saw it on the Today show, and I thought she was too young, but she isn't."

"By the time she's older, the technology should be phenomenal," Jen said.

"This generation, it amazes me what you go through," Stacy's sister Leslie said. "All my friends had three and four kids and we never had all this."

"All these chemicals," Jen said.

"At least now they have treatment," Leslie said. Jen said that in Jack's case, he probably wouldn't have survived years ago. Jen reminded Stacy about starting a CaringBridge page for Katie. CaringBridge was a Web site that allowed parents of sick children to create a running journal-like report of their children's progress while at the hospital; relatives and friends could check in on Katie's page and send messages to Stacy and Steve in the hospital.

"How's Cal with everything going on lately?" Lisa asked.

"He's good with everything going on right now," Stacy said.

"I think he's going to be crying for you guys," said Kathy Trebing, Stacy's mother-in-law, who would be watching the kids for a chunk of the time while Katie was in the hospital.

"Call one of us and we'll come get him," Lisa told Kathy. "I took this entire semester off so I could be there. You know he'd love to stay over here and have a sleepover with Brandon."

"Grace was seven when Jack went in for his transplant," Jen said, referring to Jack's older sister. "She was being very strong the whole time, and then when we came home it all came out."

On February 22, the day scheduled for the liver biopsy, Katie had a cold. The surgery was postponed until March 8, which meant the start of chemo would be bumped back a week later as well. That gave Stacy and Steve the chance to attend the fund-raiser on the night of March 4.

25

"Being a Mom Is the Coolest Gift"

On Saturday evening, March 4, 2006, every spot in the parking lot of the Moose Lodge in Mount Sinai, New York, was filled.

Welcome to an Evening of Hope and Inspiration for Katie Trebing, read programs on round tables inside the lodge. Lavender balloons—Katie's favorite color—floated in the room. Friends and family of Stacy and Steve wearing SHOW ME THE MONEY buttons peddled chances to win vacations to Ireland and the Caribbean. Flowerpots with *Katie* painted on them sat on tables, a picture of Katie sticking out of each one instead of a flower.

One of the first people to arrive was James Stelling, the fertility doctor who had extracted Stacy's eggs and implanted Christopher's embryo more than eighteen months before. Two nurses from Stelling's office came as well. So did friends from Stacy's mother's motor-home club, college buddies Steve hadn't seen in years, and teachers from Katie's preschool. Nearly four hundred raffle tickets—at fifty dollars each—sold quickly, raising nearly twenty thousand dollars.

Throughout the night, formal programming was interspersed with DJ music. Members of the Trebing family spoke on stage. "Thank you very much for your support of our granddaughter," said Rich Trebing, Steve's dad, with tears streaming down his face. Steve's mom, Kathy, stood next to him wearing a Home Depot apron with pockets to collect money, raffle tickets hanging like a garland around her neck.

Stacy's friend Michelle Weinkauf spoke next: "We have received hundreds of letters. Strangers have gone out of their way to send their donations and their prayers to Katie. We have truly felt the human spirit as it shines big."

To the music of "Butterfly Kisses," a slide show began, showing pictures of Katie playing in the snow with Calvin interspersed with pictures of Katie getting blood transfusions.

Stacy's mom had her arm around Steve's mom. Stacy's dad hovered nearby. Steve's sister, Nancy, was crying. Even Steve, who had vowed not to break down, was wiping his eyes. The Trebing children were home with a babysitter.

The evening was a financial success. The money would help pay for repeated trips to Memorial Sloan-Kettering Cancer Center in Manhattan, co-pays for drugs and hospitalization, and an advanced air-filter system for the house for when Katie came home and had to be germ free. There was possibly even enough to help Katie one day have PGD herself to ensure that none of her children would be born with Diamond Blackfan anemia.

But it also was a beautiful send-off as Steve and Stacy entered the most perilous part of their battle to heal Katie.

At six forty in the morning on Wednesday, March 8, 2006, Memorial Sloan-Kettering was quiet. The indoor pediatric playroom wasn't open yet; appointments hadn't started for the day. Stacy and Steve arrived with Katie for her liver biopsy and ovary removal.

The nurses gave Stacy and Steve a hospital gown and a matching robe for them to put on Katie. Katie held on to her pink stuffed pig she'd brought with her from home. Katie had gotten a second haircut before the fund-raiser on Saturday, so her hair was now cropped to her shoulders.

Katie was assigned a bed, and Stacy and Steve drew the curtain to change her. "This is pretty," Stacy said of the hospital gown.

"I don't want to," Katie said.

"You have to put this special dress on," Stacy said.

"Why?" Katie asked.

"Because that's how they have to do your boo-boo today. Now tuck your chin," Stacy said.

"Don't put it on, don't put it on," said Katie.

A nurse came in.

"Mom, what is Kathleen having done today?" she asked.

"Liver biopsy and ovarian removal," Stacy said.

The nurse, Danielle Gehshan, asked Stacy a string of routine questions. "Any allergies? Anything to eat or drink since midnight? Any coughing, sneezing, or fever last night?"

Then she addressed Katie.

"You don't have any jewelry on, right?"

Stacy answered. "We took the jewelry off."

"You took all your makeup off this morning?" Gehshan deadpanned to Katie.

Katie nodded.

"She has a little nail polish on. Is that okay?" Stacy asked.

"Yes. It's blue, huh?" Gehshan said.

Katie watched *Power Rangers* on TV.

"Okay, pumpkin, I'm just going to put the noodle on your arm. Then you show me a big muscle, okay?" Gehshan said. She had to put the IV in so they could administer Katie's anesthesia. "Can you squeeze my finger nice and tight? Tighter. Tight, tight, tight. Nice veins. My friend Connie is just going to hold your arm nice and straight for me."

"What do you want to sing?" Stacy asked Katie. " 'Go Go, Power Rangers'? Or 'Barbara Ann'?"

" 'Barbara Ann.' "

" 'Barbara Ann' is our usual," Stacy told the nurses. "I hope you guys know 'Barbara Ann.' "

"Okay, sweetie. Quick pinch," Gehshan said.

" 'Went to the dance, looking for romance,' " Stacy sang. Steve was hovering behind them, rubbing Katie's leg. Katie was crying but she stayed still and left her arm extended.

Dr. Boulad stopped in. "How is the other hero?" he asked, meaning Christopher.

"Okay," Steve answered.

As they waited for Katie to be wheeled into surgery, Steve made magenta Play-Doh sculptures and Katie had to guess what they were. Katie was sitting up under the blanket and Steve was sitting on the bed too, by her feet.

"Do you know what this is?" he asked her.

"A triangle," Katie said.

"All right," Steve said. "Let's see. What about—"

"An *o*," Katie interrupted.

Steve pretended to be flabbergasted. "All right. I've got a harder one. Here's a harder one."

"A star!" Katie guessed.

"No," Steve said.

"A tree," Katie said.

"No," Steve said. "It's a *k*."

"For Katie!" Katie said.

"Okay, they're here for you," interrupted a nurse at about eight thirty. An orderly in a blue shower cap and scrubs pushed Katie's bed toward the operating room as Steve and Stacy walked alongside it. Katie was lying with the blanket up to her neck and Piggy next to her. "You get to ride. It's like a magic carpet," Stacy said.

"I want Daddy," Katie said.

"I'm right here. I'm not leaving," Steve said.

They got in the elevator to go to the surgical floor.

Stacy held Katie as the doctors administered anesthesia through her IV. Katie cried, "It burns," and then was out. The doctors wheeled Katie into surgery and told Steve and Stacy to come back to recovery in forty-five minutes. The Trebings headed to the cafeteria for breakfast and waited.

———————

At ten twenty, when Katie wasn't even in recovery yet, Dr. Oktay breezed through the door of the nearby New York–Presbyterian/ Weill Cornell Medical Center carrying her left ovary in a plastic container. He took it to room 405, marked LABORATORY in red letters.

Two other scientists moved quickly to cover the counter with a blue plastic liner and lay out two Styrofoam trays, each filled with crushed ice. Oktay and his assistant Ozgur Oktem put on surgical masks, gloves and shower caps. They would be working within what Oktay called "kissing distance" of the ovary, and that meant they had to be fanatical about germs.

Oktay removed three sterile petri dishes. He put a cleanser in two of them to wash the ovary. Another assistant, Gulnaz Sahin, opened one sterile bag containing scissors, and another with a scalpel. Oktay placed them both on the counter. He used sterile tweezers to remove the ovary from the container. It looked like a pink lima bean. An adult ovary is normally the size of a walnut. "You cannot just freeze the tissue like you put food in your freezer or the eggs will not survive," Oktay explained as he worked.

Oktay swished it around in the petri dish. He then moved the ovary to a second dish of wash. Next, working very delicately with a scalpel, he began to remove the connective tissue surrounding the ovary. For thirty minutes, Oktay trimmed the ovary; its texture was like an unripe plum. He didn't have to worry about "breaking" eggs; they weren't as fragile as hen's eggs, and they were embedded in the tissue.

"I'm getting ready to make the final trim and we're going to cut it in tiny pieces," Oktay told his assistants. He proceeded, slicing the ovary with his scalpel into tiny slivers each the size of a grain of rice.

The thinness of the slices was critical because a medical antifreeze substance had to penetrate the tissue before it was frozen or ice crystals would form during the freezing process. Their sharp edges could damage the eggs. Oktay picked up each sliver with the tweezers and placed it into a vial of medical antifreeze. He had to shake the tweezers to get the piece of ovary to drop off.

Oktay put the small vials into long tubes filled with ice. Then the tubes were rolled in more ice for half an hour so the antifreeze could penetrate the tissue from all sides; the ovary slice sloshed around in each vial like laundry in the washing machine. The vials were then frozen slowly over the span of three hours.

They would be stored until Katie—decades later—was ready to have children. When the strips were implanted in Katie, they would fuse back together. "The ovary is one of the most malleable organs in the body," Oktay said.

Katie Trebing was believed to be the youngest girl ever to have an ovary removed and frozen for future use. Ovarian cryopreservation had been done for about a decade. In 2002, the year Katie was born, Oktay froze an ovary for Ann Dauer, who was then twenty-nine and needed a stem cell transplant to survive non-Hodgkin's lymphoma. In 2005, after her ovary was reimplanted, she gave birth to a baby girl.

"Being a mom is the coolest gift you can ever get," said Dauer, who lives in Cincinnati. Being able to freeze her ovary gave Dauer hope during her battle to survive. She was told a stem cell transplant would give her a 30 percent chance of surviving the disease; she made the decision to go ahead with the transplant, but she also asked the doctors if it would affect her fertility. "The oncologist at Sloan was probably thinking, 'This girl's crazy. She has a thirty percent chance she's going to beat this and she's talking about fertility?'" But the oncologist was a woman with five children, so she understood. She put Dauer in touch with Dr. Oktay. After her ovary was removed and frozen, Dauer said she would lie in the hospital bed thinking, *I've done every step I can to keep all my dreams alive.*

After Dauer's lymphoma was successfully cured by the transplant and she was ready to have children, her ovary was reimplanted in her body. In Dauer's case, Oktay reimplanted it in her groin, beneath the skin between her belly button and pubic bone.

He fanned the ovary strips out like a deck of cards so there'd be more surface area to extract eggs from. Dauer started hormone shots and could feel little bumps of eggs developing under her skin. Oktay had planned to extract eggs with a needle and do in vitro fertilization.

But when he did an exam prior to withdrawing her eggs, Dauer remembers Oktay saying, "Oh my God, oh my God, oh my God."

"I'm thinking, 'What happened to the ovary?' I'm thinking it disintegrated. He said, 'You're pregnant.' I'm like, 'What are you talking about? How did that happen?'" Dauer's chemotherapy before her bone marrow transplant had put her into early menopause, as expected. Oktay theorized that the transplanted ovary tissue "jump-started" the ovary left in place inside Dauer, taking her out of premature menopause and restoring fertility. That first pregnancy miscarried at six weeks, but Dauer started to menstruate and got pregnant again naturally with a daughter she named Sienna. She has since had a second baby naturally, Gregory Jr., born in February of 2009.

The perfection of ovarian cryopreservation and subsequent reimplantation is important to many women diagnosed with cancer, blood diseases, or other disorders that require radiation and chemotherapy, which can cause infertility. If they can have an ovary removed before the eggs are damaged, they might later have biological children.

Oktay found it disturbing that while doctors could cure a woman of cancer, they would leave her infertile. "It didn't make sense to me that while we were treating a woman for one thing, we would leave her severely disabled—and infertility is a disability," Oktay opined. Oktay was also working on ways to protect women's ovaries during chemotherapy to eliminate the need for ovary removal.

By the day of Katie's surgery, Oktay had removed and frozen ovaries from about ninety women, though none as young as Katie. He called ovarian cryopreservation a "burgeoning technology."

Though ovarian cryopreservation was meant for cancer patients, it could in the future open up opportunities for all women—a healthy woman who wanted to delay childbirth could have an ovary frozen while she was still young and fertile, suspending the aging of the eggs.

"If our method works, a young woman age twenty-one and entering law school or journalism school or medical school could cryopreserve her ovary for later use," said Teresa Woodruff, the Thomas J. Watkins Professor of Obstetrics and Gynecology at the Feinberg School of Medicine at Northwestern University in Chicago. "Rather than take a chance with the biological clock, you could cryopreserve your ovary and use it when you are ready. You would be your own egg donor."

While doctors had advanced the freezing technique, they were still working on the best way to reimplant the ovary so that it might enable a pregnancy years down the road. Woodruff and her team, on the other hand, were working on maturing the eggs from previously cryopreserved ovaries in the laboratory. The matured eggs would then be fertilized in a petri dish and the embryo implanted into the woman's womb, as in IVF. In this case, the benefit—in addition to eliminating the need for women to take certain fertility medications and have ovary-implantation surgery—would be that cancer patients wouldn't risk reintroducing cancerous cells into their systems along with the reimplanted ovary. In 2007, Woodruff was awarded a $21 million grant from the National Institutes of Health to continue her work on preserving fertility in cancer patients.

As with all innovative medical technologies, there is an element of the unknown in ovarian cryopreservation that concerns some bioethicists.

When individuals try most new treatments, they are risking only their own health. But when they try new reproductive technologies, they impose that risk on their offspring, said Alta Charo, professor of law and bioethics at the University of Wisconsin. No data yet exists on implications for a child born of a frozen ovary. "When you, the adult, accept there is risk, it's really your child who will share the burden of those risks," Charo said. But for couples like the Dauers, who have two apparently healthy children, the chance to raise a family seems to outweigh all the ethical issues.

Steve and Stacy were by Katie's side when she woke up in recovery, groggy and cranky. For the rest of the day, Katie was in so much pain that Stacy questioned whether she'd be a strong enough mother to watch her daughter go through the bone marrow transplant ordeal. Although removing one of Katie's ovaries appeared to give Katie the best chance of having children in the future, Stacy felt sorrow that a surgeon had removed a part of her little girl. Stacy slept overnight next to Katie's bed, and by the next morning Katie was feeling better. They all went home so that they'd be there on Friday, March 10, to celebrate Calvin's sixth birthday. Katie slept the whole way home. She had a bandage over her belly button that would stay on for two weeks.

26

"It's Now or Never"

On Monday, March 20, Katie returned to Sloan-Kettering for pre-transplant testing. She needed an echocardiogram to make sure that at the start of transplant her heart function was normal, and the doctors did a DNA test using a swab of the inside of Katie's mouth. That swab showed, among other things, that Katie had *not* developed a sensitivity to little e. The initial finding that she had was actually an error. Katie also had a blood test to make sure she didn't have any viruses in her system that could flare up during the chemotherapy and kill her.

Though they'd been prepared for the possibility, the Trebings were nonetheless stunned that day to learn that Dr. Boulad was no longer open to using Christopher's cord blood and definitely wanted to use his actual bone marrow instead. He believed that would better Katie's chances.

That meant Christopher also had to come into the hospital for pretransplant blood workups.

Two days later, the Trebings got more disconcerting news. Dr. Boulad called with the results of Katie's liver biopsy. Her iron content was a 3-plus on a scale of 4, higher than they had hoped. The scarring to the liver was a 1 on the same scale, which was encouraging. And there was an additional issue. Before the Trebings found out that Katie shouldn't receive blood donations from family members, Steve's mom had donated blood for her. The Trebings thought they were doing the right thing, but that move could possibly have caused Katie to develop antibodies to her grandmother's DNA. Boulad had ordered Steve's mom tested to see if she shared any markers with Christopher; it turned out she was a half DNA match to him. Therefore, Boulad would have to add another chemotherapy drug called cyclophosphamide, sold under the brand name Cytoxan, to Katie's regimen. This could be more toxic to her liver, increasing her chances of developing veno-occlusive disease, which could fatally shut down her liver. The Trebings were distraught. Stacy wanted to know whether the transplant was still the best choice for Katie, given this new information. Dr. Boulad assured her that while he was a transplant doctor, he was a human being first and would never put a child in the way of unnecessary harm. It was still, in his opinion, Katie's best shot at a long and healthy life.

On Friday Christopher had to come to Sloan-Kettering to be tested again, and the blood test was just as difficult and draining as the first time. The nurses stuck him unsuccessfully seven times before Dr. Kobos had to come in and take Christopher's blood through a vein in his foot. And it turned out that the testing was wasted— Katie's blood tests came back showing a parasite that she'd probably picked up playing in the dirt in the backyard. This would delay the start of the bone marrow procedure for four weeks.

On April 19 Katie and Christopher went through their pre-admission testing again. Any health issues for Katie had to be cleared up prior to transplant, and now she needed to have a cavity filled. Katie was frantic as the pediatric dentist attempted to work on her. She was kicking, crying, and inconsolable. The dentist told Steve that filling the cavity would take only three minutes, and it had to be done because it could prove a route to infection during the transplant. So Steve pushed away his guilt and helped put Katie into what looked to him like a straitjacket. They then secured Katie, lying down, to a gurney. As the dentist reached for his tools, Katie's eyes widened. She vomited in fear and started to choke.

Instinctively, Steve grabbed the gurney and turned it on its side. Medical tools flew into the air as the assistant's tray tipped over. Katie spit out the vomit and gasped for air. Steve unstrapped the Velcro holding Katie, and she lunged toward him and wrapped her arms around his neck in a vise grip. They gave up, and Stacy told Dr. Boulad what had happened. Boulad arranged for Katie to have the cavity filled while she was under general anesthesia having her central line put in her chest.

On April 27, Katie had her central line placed in anticipation of her checking into Sloan-Kettering for her bone marrow transplant on May 1. The Trebings' insurance company had given them approval to go ahead. Katie seemed excited to have her central line attached. Stacy felt like her preschooler knew this was her chance to get better and wanted it to happen already.

But on Monday, May 1, Katie woke up with a runny nose. Even though Stacy had hugged Calvin and Christopher and kissed them good-bye as if she'd be leaving for the next month, the Trebings were sent back home to wait again.

It was another emotional letdown. They drove back to Nesconset and unpacked for another week. Stacy would have to keep Katie inside to get her better. No playdates, no mall, no trips to the movies to pass the time. Even in the house, Stacy would have to keep the three kids away from one another as much as possible so nobody infected anybody else. Even Katie seemed disappointed.

For Steve, the continued delay was a nightmare. "It's the busiest six weeks of the year," he said. "June is chock-full of weddings and graduations." The only good part was the whole family was home when Christopher turned one, on May 4, 2006.

On May 8, Katie was sent home again because she still had the remnants of a cold.

The Trebings tried again on the morning of May 15, more than two months after the original target date. For Stacy, the trip seemed anticlimactic. The night before, Stacy had attempted some humor in a post on the CaringBridge page she'd created for Katie. She'd been surfing the Web and had found a list called "You Know

Your Child Is Getting a Transplant When…" She copied it onto Katie's page, changing a few items to make it apply especially to her daughter.

Number 3: When asked which kid is yours on the playground, you say, "The bald one."

Number 5: Your child has thrown up twice in one day, and you smile at what a good day it has been.

And number 8: When the siblings think Mommy and Daddy live at the Ronald McDonald House and Katie lives in the hospital.

In the morning, Stacy had to call the oil company to schedule a delivery as she finished packing up Katie's shorts and T-shirts and pajamas for the hospital. For the third time she hugged Calvin and Christopher, expecting that she wouldn't see them for at least a week, depending on how she and Steve split up the time by Katie's bedside. It would be the longest she'd ever been apart from the boys. Cal left for school, and Steve's parents arrived to babysit for Christopher.

A teeming rain fell gloomy and gray as Stacy and Steve drove Katie into Manhattan. "It's now or never," Steve said to himself as they left Nesconset. They stopped at a BJ's Wholesale Club, the local shopping warehouse store, because Stacy wanted to buy a portable DVD player for their time in the hospital. Stacy asked the woman behind the checkout counter to cut it out of the heavy plastic container.

"Are you going on a road trip?" the saleswoman asked Katie. "You are so lucky. Where are you going?"

Stacy couldn't resist a little mischief.

"She's going to get a bone marrow transplant at Memorial Sloan-Kettering Cancer Center," Stacy responded.

The clerk appeared mortified.

"Oh, good luck," she said.

On the drive to the Upper East Side, Katie watched *Cinderella*. She wore a light blue hat that was decorated with butterfly and ladybug pins and had *Katie* written on it in purple script. Steve's aunt Kathy had given it to her so she could wear it when her hair fell out. She told Katie it was a "huggable" hat. "Every time you need a hug, put the hat on and we'll be hugging you," she said.

Stacy felt it was a good sign when she noticed that the church on East Sixty-eighth Street, across from the hospital, was St. Catherine of Siena, the same name as the Long Island hospital where her children were born.

Steve dropped off Stacy and Katie in front of the hospital. Katie pulled her Bitty Baby American Girl suitcase into the hospital, rolling it behind her like the hospital pro she was. The Trebings reported to the ninth floor and were assigned what would be Katie's room for the next six weeks, the room where her future would be decided.

Room 935.

27

"Bubba's My Brother"

A bone marrow transplant has three phases while the patient is in the hospital. The first phase lasts ten days, during which doctors count down from Day Negative Ten to Day Zero. During that first phase, Katie would get chemotherapy drugs to wipe out her immune system. The second phase was just one day long: Day Zero, the day Christopher would be brought into Sloan-Kettering. His marrow would be removed and then transferred into Katie. The third phase was post-transplant, when the doctors waited for Christopher's marrow to start making red blood cells in Katie and for Katie's immune system to grow strong enough for her to be released from the hospital. Every day of the third phase would be counted in positive numbers—Day One, Day Two—for the four more weeks Katie would likely spend in Memorial Sloan-Kettering. The most dangerous period for Katie would be the first two weeks after Day Zero, but serious risks could linger for up to a hundred days.

MONDAY, MAY 15, 2006: DAY NEGATIVE TEN

The first thing Stacy did was decorate. Stacy hung construction paper get-well cards created for Katie by a local school class that had read about Katie's upcoming transplant in a newspaper. She put up a string of decorative lights with tiny lampshades in pinks and purples and plaid she had bought on clearance at Target. On the window ledge she set a snow globe with an angel in it that Stacy's mom had given to Katie. Next to it went a statue of Saint Theresa that Stacy's friend Adrienne Law had given her.

Stacy set a little blue angel next to the telephone. Katie had told Stacy that she'd had a dream about a blue angel who watched over all sick children. Stacy felt Katie was speaking of Stacy's maternal grandmother. Stacy had been very close to her grandmother Mimi and missed her terribly. Mimi had passed away when Stacy was pregnant with Calvin, so Mimi never got to meet any of Stacy's children. Mimi had worn a blue dress to Stacy and Steve's wedding, and five years later, when she died, she was buried in that same blue dress.

Despite the decorations Stacy brought, there was no masking the fact that this was a hospital room. Medical equipment hung on a wall behind Katie's bed. Katie's grown-up twin hospital bed had crisp, white sheets, pillows, and blankets. A coatrack-like IV stand was hooked to the central line previously inserted in Katie's chest; Katie would be attached to the rolling IV stand until the day she left Memorial Sloan-Kettering. At the peak of Katie's treatment, the stand would be holding a dozen bags filled with drugs and liquids. Stacy and Katie decided to nickname the IV stand Bubble Buddy, after a character in a *SpongeBob* episode, since it was like another person in the room with them.

Katie remembered the hospital from her liver biopsy and ovary removal, which proved both a good and bad thing. She remembered that the bed vibrated periodically to prevent the patient from getting bed sores, and that had annoyed her, so she didn't want to get on the bed.

More happily, Katie also remembered the inpatient playroom—a smaller play area for bone marrow patients—filled with toys she could bring back to her hospital room. Katie was allowed in there in the days prior to being put into isolation, and she made a beeline to collect her loot, choosing a Magna Doodle and a puzzle. Soon Katie would be prohibited from touching any games that any other child had touched, for fear of her picking up germs.

The doctors began to visit in what to Stacy seemed like herds. They weren't sugarcoating anything: they reminded Stacy to prepare for Katie's nausea, mouth sores, and loss of appetite. They told her to let Katie eat whatever she wanted for now because they expected she would eventually lose weight. The chemotherapy would temporarily kill off her taste buds and they would take a few months to return. Right away they started the drug Dilantin through Katie's IV line; it was an antiseizure medication the doctors gave in advance before they started the chemotherapy drug busulfan, which could cause seizures.

The Dilantin made Katie loopy. Stacy thought Katie was acting like a girl in her freshman year at college experimenting with alcohol. It was comical at first, but then Katie's behavior got very difficult, and she stayed restless until finally falling asleep at nine thirty that night. Steve went home after that, because the city's nearby Ronald McDonald House, which offered inexpensive rooms to families whose children were hospitalized, was booked for the week.

A nurse and Stacy had to wake Katie up throughout the night to swallow liquid doses of one drug to help prevent pneumonia and another to prevent the herpes virus. They had to hold Katie down and force her to take it. Stacy was surprised that they started so many medicines already, on Katie's first night.

The first week wouldn't be so bad, Stacy knew. It would be the second and third week when Katie would have nausea, diarrhea, and mouth sores. It would be even longer before Katie lost her hair. The other moms whose children had already been through chemotherapy told Stacy the hair loss wouldn't be as disconcerting as she probably imagined. "With all the other things going on, who gives a crap about hair?" they pointed out.

TUESDAY, MAY 16, 2006: DAY NEGATIVE NINE

Steve came back in the morning, and he and Stacy took turns playing Pretty Pretty Princess, Connect Four, and I Spy with Katie to keep her busy. They watched movies and TV. Katie didn't have to wear a hospital gown; she was in blue jeans and a long-sleeved pink shirt with flowers on the front. Her hair was in a short bob with bangs.

To pass the time, Stacy read gossip magazines like *Star*, losing herself in stories about Brad Pitt and Angelina Jolie. Sometimes Steve would pick up one of Stacy's magazines and page through until Katie noticed what he was reading and admonished him, saying, "Dad, those magazines are for girls." Stacy also started *The Purpose Driven Life*, a spiritual book that promised to explain God's purpose for one's life. Readers were supposed to tackle one chapter each day for forty days; Stacy thought it would be a good way to mark the passage of time.

The busulfan protocol had begun. Stacy and Steve had to catch all of Katie's urine and feces in a basin in the toilet; at night Katie had to wear a special diaper. The doctors tested Katie's waste to see how Katie's body was handling the medications.

Stacy slept overnight on a recliner next to Katie's hospital bed. Stacy had brought a white-noise machine to the hospital to help her sleep, but the beeping from Katie's IV pole still woke her up two or three times a night. Sometimes the IV machine beeped because a medication had finished; sometimes it was because a kink had formed in the IV line. Stacy would call a nurse, who would come to adjust it. In time, Stacy would learn to adjust it herself.

WEDNESDAY, MAY 17: DAY NEGATIVE EIGHT

Katie still had her normal energy, though she was dizzy from the Dilantin. She often forgot she had the IV pole connected to her and took off for the inpatient playroom with Stacy or Steve following behind, pushing the pole and screaming, "Stop!" They had to restrict Katie from moving around too fast.

Katie also had mood swings caused by the Dilantin—happy at one moment and then viciously screaming "I hate you" at Steve, Stacy, the nurses, anyone who came into her orbit.

Katie wasn't in any pain so far because everything was administered orally or through her IV tubes. The hardest part for her seemed to be missing Calvin and Christopher and wanting to go home to Nesconset. Katie could call home and talk on a video phone that was in Steve and Stacy's bedroom. But it was hard to do. Steve's parents had moved into the younger Trebings' house to take care of Calvin and Christopher; on their end, Christopher was always trying to grab the phone, and Calvin got a little crazy. He would stick his tongue out, or make faces. Stacy and Katie made a colorful paper chain with a number on each loop; it started at −8 and went through 0 and then up to 20. They hung the chain from the ceiling. This was a suggestion from a DBA patient in Florida who had also had a bone marrow transplant: each ring represented a day Katie spent in the hospital, and Stacy and Katie would remove a ring every night so Katie could visualize her time at Sloan-Kettering getting shorter and shorter. Stacy realized twenty-eight rings was an unreasonably low number—it should be closer to forty—but more than twenty-eight just looked too overwhelming. She would add numbers in a few nights, while Katie was sleeping.

Nurses brought the Trebings some disconcerting news. Dr. Boulad—the teddy bear of a doctor they had chosen to do Christopher's bone marrow extraction and Katie's transplant—had experienced a family tragedy. His mother had died, and he had to travel back to Lebanon immediately for her funeral. He would be gone for ten days. Instead of Boulad, another doctor, Nancy Kernan, attending physician of Sloan-Kettering's pediatric bone marrow transplant service, would perform Christopher's bone marrow retrieval as well as Katie's transplant.

That rattled the Trebings, but what could they do? Katie had already started the chemotherapy regimen. The staff assured them that Dr. Kernan was an excellent doctor who had conferred in detail with Dr. Boulad about Katie and Christopher.

That night, when a nurse came in to give Katie medicine, Stacy explained to Katie a little bit about Christopher. "That's the medicine that's going to get rid of the bad blood. Bubba is going to give you his blood," Stacy said.

"Is Bubba sick?" Katie asked.

"No, he has good blood."

"Who's Bubba?" the nurse asked.

"Bubba's my brother," Katie replied.

THURSDAY, MAY 18: DAY NEGATIVE SEVEN

Katie was adjusting to life at the hospital. Instead of having to be held down to take her medicine, like on the first night, Katie happily slurped it up and then licked the inside of the cup. The hospital used cherry flavoring to make the medicine more appealing. "I wish every patient was like this," one nurse said.

Stacy and Steve noticed that Katie's breath and urine smelled like the chemotherapy drugs. "Poison flowing into her" was how Stacy sometimes saw it, reminding her of the steroids. She found it ironic that in her normal parenting life, she didn't even like to give her children chemicals as mild as food coloring, yet here she was allowing doctors to flood her daughter with potentially toxic drugs.

Steve went home tonight, I am so jealous that he gets to see the boys, Stacy posted on Katie's page on the CaringBridge site, using the laptop she'd brought to the hospital so she could write daily entries and put up photos of Katie. *I miss the hugs!! I wonder what Christopher will do when I come home, I try to remember that lots of parents have to be apart from their kids for various reasons and it all works out. Steve will come back to the hospital on Sunday and I will go home to be with the boys until Monday. Thanks for all of the notes and prayers.* Stacy would often sign her entries, *From the Inside.*

Before going to sleep, Katie and Stacy took a ring off the paper chain.

FRIDAY, MAY 19: DAY NEGATIVE SIX

The list of intravenous medications was daunting. Katie finished the busulfan regimen and started on a drug called fludarabine, which would render her immune system powerless so it wouldn't reject Christopher's bone marrow. It would also leave Katie temporarily defenseless against infection.

Stacy had moments when she thought about life being normal and being out at Steve's parents' house on the beach in Fire Island. But it was too late; they couldn't turn back. They had begun to shut down Katie's immune system in preparation for the transplant; if they stopped the process now, Katie would definitely die.

The hospital stay was getting tedious for Stacy, who had been there round the clock for five days already. It was difficult to live the life of a three-year-old day after day, playing endless games of bingo, going back and forth with Katie to the small playroom meant only for bone marrow inpatients who hadn't yet lost all immunity, then to her hospital room, then to the playroom, then to her hospital room, trying to keep Katie entertained. On one trip to the playroom, Katie played with Play-Doh, but each canister had to be newly opened and played with by only one patient and then thrown away to prevent the spread of germs. "I hate you!" Katie yelled at the black Play-Doh when she couldn't get the lid open. Katie drew crayon pictures—one she said was "a worm sleeping." Another was "a snail blowing air."

Suddenly Katie said to Stacy, "I want to go home."

"You want to go back to your room?" Stacy clarified.

"No, I want to go home, I want to see Cal. I want to see Daddy," Katie said.

This was when Stacy had to become a master of distraction. "We have to stay a little while longer. The candy cart is coming tonight. You can pick candy." A cart came to each child's room every Friday evening filled with M&Ms, Twizzlers, and other treats, and children could take as much candy as they wanted. Katie had been looking forward to her first visit from the candy cart.

Back in her room, Katie finger painted, the purple paint staining all the way up her forearms. And she played hide-and-seek with Stacy, crawling underneath the pillows on her bed, her pink slippers with the bunny heads on them sometimes sticking out from underneath. Katie's hospital room was looking more lived in. A sign on the door said KATIE'S ROOM. A picture Calvin had made hung on the wall.

Stacy had made Katie a doll with an IV that went into her chest, just like Katie had. Katie's dressing had to be cleaned every few days; Katie would pretend she was cleaning the doll's central line as well. She would sometimes sit for half an hour doing that.

Once in a while, someone from Child Life, the hospital department that supported the parents in keeping their offspring as happy as possible, would knock on Katie's door. Today it was the clown Dr. Keyspan and his sidekick Dr. Quackenbush. "No relation to the president," Dr. Quackenbush said cheerily. He had a big red nose, green sneakers, and a yellow hat.

"Can I tell you a secret?" Katie asked Stacy. That's what she said when she didn't want to hurt someone's feelings. Stacy leaned down so Katie could whisper in her ear. "I want them to go away." She wasn't in the mood for strangers.

Other times, Katie was friendly.

A nurse came in to work with Katie's IV lines.

"What are you doing?" Katie asked her.

"I'm flushing your tube," she said.

"That's my new friend," Katie told her mom. When the nurse left, Katie pretended to take blood from a visitor. She had her own syringe filled with saline solution that the nurses gave her. She took out an alcohol pad to rub the mock patient's arm. "This won't hurt," Katie said. "It's going to feel a little cold. Keep your arm froze. Don't move. We have to do this so you don't get an infection."

Stacy worked constantly to fight germs. If a pillow fell on the floor, she changed the pillowcase. If a crayon fell on the floor, she swiped it with an antibacterial wipe before she let Katie touch it again. She reminded Katie repeatedly not to put her hands in her mouth. She couldn't cut Katie's nails because a nick would open a site to infection; she had to use a nail file to shorten them. Soon, Katie wouldn't be allowed to brush her teeth for the same reason and would instead use a creamy antifungal mouth rinse.

If a child coughed in the playroom, Stacy worried the germ might reach Katie. If the front desk got a flower delivery, Stacy worried because fresh flowers carry bacteria. Every time Katie sneezed, Stacy worried she'd caught a cold that could kill her.

Another nurse came in.

"Did you wash your hands?" Stacy asked.

"They're still wet," the nurse replied.

At home in Nesconset, Steve's parents had been going through their own ordeal keeping one-year-old Christopher healthy. They had to keep him away from other children. Katie needed Christopher's marrow on schedule, and if he contracted an infection, he'd pass it on to her and she might not be able to withstand it.

SATURDAY, MAY 20: DAY NEGATIVE FIVE

Katie had had a tough day; she'd finally gotten the nausea and discomfort the doctors had warned about. It broke Stacy's heart that she couldn't do anything to make her daughter feel better.

After Katie was asleep, Stacy watched her frail-looking daughter, hooked up to so many tubes. She was lying next to Katie on Katie's bed. She wanted to call Steve, but debated whether it was too late. She worried about the phone's ring waking up Calvin and Christopher. But she needed her husband badly. She dialed.

Stacy was crying so much she could hardly talk. Steve rarely let himself think about Katie's dying, but Stacy sometimes imagined it. Watching the drugs flow into Katie and not knowing what might happen was too much for Stacy to bear alone. The unknown was terrifying.

SUNDAY, MAY 21: DAY NEGATIVE FOUR

Steve arrived early Sunday to relieve Stacy so she could spend a night home with the boys prior to Katie's transplant. Steve was nervous that Katie could only be comforted by her mom, but he came prepared to give it his best shot. For most of the day, Steve had one job: be a clown. He made funny noises and goofy laughs, took pretend falls, and did anything else he could think of to make his daughter laugh. *Today was harder than any day I ever had at work,* Steve thought.

The low point of the day came at four o'clock, when doctors gave Katie a dose of the chemotherapy drug Cytoxan, the extra drug she had to take because Steve's mother had once donated blood to her. Katie became extremely nauseated for about two hours. *This is nasty stuff,* Steve thought. Katie also got another drug to increase her fluid output. Steve took Katie to the bathroom what felt like thirty-five times in a few hours, changing her whenever she accidentally soaked her pajamas.

Back at home, Stacy read Steve's CaringBridge entry about his day with Katie, and added her own comment. *It's times like this when you truly fall in love again, for all different reasons,* she wrote.

MONDAY, MAY 22: DAY NEGATIVE THREE

Katie was still miserable; sleepy and drained and moody. Steve had gotten up with her five times during the night to take her to the bathroom. "Why doesn't she complain?" Steve marveled. He, on the other hand, was tempted to whine. The doctors had enacted Katie's isolation, and now Steve had to wear a yellow paper gown, latex gloves, and a white surgical mask in Katie's room at all times to protect Katie from potential germs. Steve thought it was hot and confining in the room, and there was no way to open the windows.

Katie got more chemotherapy drugs. She got one called Rabbit ATG, or anti-thymocyte globulin, purified from the serum of rabbits. It would kill Katie's T cells. Shortly after it was administered, Katie's fever spiked. Her body shivered uncontrollably, and it seemed to Steve as if Katie were outside in a snowstorm without a jacket. If the doctors hadn't warned Steve about the side effects, he would have panicked. Instead, he just tried to make Katie as comfortable as possible.

Katie wanted to throw up, and Steve grabbed a yellow bucket and aimed it under her chin just in time. As Katie was dry heaving and phlegm was dripping off her lips, Steve was relieved to hear her yell, "Dad, moooove!" He was blocking her view of the television set. How bad could she be if she was still worried about watching her cartoons?

TUESDAY, MAY 23: DAY NEGATIVE TWO

Stacy drove back to Sloan-Kettering along with her parents and Christopher because Christopher had to have presurgery blood testing in anticipation of Thursday's transplant procedure. Stacy stayed with Katie, while Steve and her parents went with Christopher for his blood test.

Stacy felt her emotions welling up. She suddenly realized that she still had Christopher's diaper bag with her; her dad had taken one of her bags instead. She called him on his cell phone. "Dad, you're giving me a heart attack," she said. "Do you have my bag?"

Just then, the medical team walked in. Stacy felt like an idiot. Here she was going nuts over a missing bag when her daughter was on the verge of a bone marrow transplant. When her father walked back to exchange bags with her, Stacy burst into tears.

Again the nurses had problems drawing Christopher's blood. They tried six times to insert a needle on one side of his body, seven times on the other. Steve was pinning Christopher down, his head on Christopher's chest. A nurse practitioner held Christopher's feet. Christopher was kicking and flailing and crying so hard he was gasping. At one point they finally managed to draw some blood, but halfway through they lost the vein and had to start all over again.

Steve looked up and saw tears coming down the nurse practitioner's face. "Don't make eye contact!" Steve yelled to her. "Don't look at his face!" The nurses gave up and called Dr. Rachel Kobos, who drew blood from an artery in Christopher's wrist, a more dangerous procedure that a physician is needed to do. As soon as Kobos was done, Steve gave Christopher a bottle and he fell asleep for an hour. Stacy's parents took Christopher back home to Nesconset.

WEDNESDAY, MAY 24: DAY NEGATIVE ONE

On Wednesday morning, hospital staff members bleached the peach-colored walls in Katie's room to kill any germs. They changed the curtains in the room, changed her bedding.

Katie would have no more chemotherapy today. To entertain her, Steve let Katie snap his latex gloves. She pulled the thumb out and let it zing back. It hurt Steve's hand, but Katie loved it, so he didn't complain. Katie didn't have to wear the protective gear, but everyone else did. She'd had a hard time with her parents wearing gowns and masks and gloves at first, and Steve was just happy she was having some fun with it. Steve wore a necklace of alphabet blocks on a string that Katie had made for him.

Katie was defenseless now; she had no immune system. That scared Stacy, even though it was the way it had to be. Katie was no longer allowed to leave her room. She had a rash and diarrhea, but that wasn't a surprise to the doctors. She also had a slight cough, so doctors took a chest X-ray, which came back normal.

Stacy's parents arrived back in Manhattan with Christopher. They would be sharing a room at the nearby Ronald McDonald House with Steve. The staff instructed Steve about preparing Christopher. He could have nothing to drink after midnight except water. He should arrive at the hospital at seven fifteen; his procedure was scheduled for nine. Stacy was happy that Steve would be the one with Christopher and her parents, for two reasons. Number one, Christopher was not going to be at all happy about being denied food. And number two, her dad snored. Stacy preferred to have Katie duty this time.

Steve and Stacy were worried about Christopher's procedure. It was stressful enough that Dr. Boulad was in Lebanon and another doctor would be subbing for him. But the doctors had also told the Trebings that they were concerned about how hard it had been to take Christopher's blood in each instance. If the doctors couldn't get an IV into Christopher's arm the next day, they would have to go through a vein in his leg, which would be more dangerous. Christopher might then have to stay overnight in the hospital. Steve and Stacy worried that would cause complications for Christopher; Stacy asked everyone reading Katie's CaringBridge page to pray for an easy time for her son.

Stacy needed a break from the hospital room before Steve

joined her parents and Christopher at the Ronald McDonald House for the night.

So Stacy yanked off the yellow paper hospital gown that covered her shorts and T-shirt, unhooked the surgical mask from behind her ears, and stuffed both items into the garbage pail in the entryway of her daughter's hospital room.

She needed that breather.

She headed to the ninth floor's family sitting area, where she sank onto a couch.

The next day would be the culmination of the Trebings' years-long journey. Many of the parents called it Rebirth Day and celebrated it every year in addition to the child's birthday. Stacy did feel almost festive, like the big day had finally arrived.

But while the journey had been focused on Katie, Stacy considered the next day was really about Christopher. It would be his big day, his big performance. Christopher was expected to cure his sister. But what if Katie's body rejected Christopher's marrow and Katie died? Would it change how Stacy felt about Christopher? Would it make it harder to be his mother? *If anything ever happened to Katie,* Stacy asked herself, *would I be resentful toward him?*

But the answer came to her quickly. *How could I be?* she thought. *Out of all this, I got Christopher.*

28

"Good Luck"

Stacy opened her eyes at seven ten that morning. She knew Christopher was supposed to be at the hospital by seven fifteen. Katie was still asleep. Stacy couldn't use the bathroom in Katie's room because it needed to be kept sterile. She pulled off her gloves, mask, and gown. Stacy didn't sleep in pajamas—she slept in clothes in case she had to use the bathroom in the middle of the night. Stacy walked down the hall to the floor's common bathroom, where she brushed her teeth and washed her face.

Then she stopped at the shared kitchen on the floor to get a cup of coffee. Three other mothers were in the pantry, other mothers whose children were in the process of bone marrow transplants. Other mothers who knew what today meant for Katie. "This is my daughter's big day," Stacy told them. "My son's coming in and he's getting his bone marrow taken."

"I'm going to prayer group right now," one mother said. "I'll pray for you."

"Good luck," a second mother simply wished.

Stacy went back to Katie's room to wait for her mom to arrive to sit with Katie so Stacy could go see Christopher before his marrow extraction. She went online to check e-mail on her laptop; her friend Michelle had e-mailed with a link to the song "Wildflowers" by Tom Petty. Stacy went to iTunes and bought it for Katie so she could hear it as she woke up.

At eight thirty, Stacy played the song and woke Katie. She still hadn't heard from Steve or her parents, but she knew that by now, they must be in the waiting area around the corner. A nurse came in. "Can I run over and see how they're doing?" Stacy asked. The nurse agreed to sit with Katie while Stacy went.

Steve and Christopher had already been up for hours. Christopher was Steve's alarm clock that morning at five thirty. Stacy's parents, Steve, and Christopher were all sleeping in the same room, with Christopher in a porta-crib next to Steve's bed. With no place to go, the four of them got up to start the day.

It was going to be beautiful; even at six thirty, the day was warm with a slight breeze. The accent lighting was still on next to the building doorways along York Avenue. The sun was coming through the side streets between the high-rise buildings, not high enough in the sky to scale them yet. The buildings threw shadows across the sidewalks. People already were crisscrossing the streets in the empire that made up New York-Presbyterian Weill Cornell Medical Center and Memorial Sloan-Kettering Cancer Center on Manhattan's Upper East Side. Some people on their way to work bought doughnuts or buttered hard rolls from the silver trucks parked along the street; many of them were wearing the distinctive white coats of medical professionals, and some were in scrubs with teddy bears on them. Steve carried Christopher to the hospital.

It was the day before the start of Memorial Day weekend, the kickoff of New York's summer season. The newspapers were filled with ads for swimsuits. Manhattan's annual Fleet Week had just started, filling the city with sailors dressed in white. Later in the day C-130 planes would swoop above Memorial Sloan-Kettering in formations of six.

Today, no clowns would visit Katie. In room 935, the day would be all about a bag of bright red liquid that would hang from Bubble Buddy, the IV rack in Katie's room, and drip slowly into Katie to try to fix what was wrong with her, to change her fate. Sister and brother would not see each other today. They would be entirely separate this day at Memorial Sloan-Kettering, except for the fact that Christopher's bone marrow would be carried over to Katie's room and transferred into her.

As soon as Stacy saw Christopher, she could tell he was cranky. He wasn't used to waiting to eat in the morning. Stacy felt like her baby was looking at her and thinking, *Where have you been?* Steve and Stacy decided to split the tasks of the day by gender. Her dad would stay with Steve and Christopher; her mom would come back with Stacy to Katie's room. Stacy's mom was glad she was at the hospital, knowing what was happening to her grandchildren all day, rather than home on Long Island, waiting for telephone updates like the rest of the family.

This was Pam Olsen's first visit to see her granddaughter at Sloan-Kettering, and she was hesitant to enter Katie's room. She put on the gown, mask, and gloves and steeled herself. She found it heartbreaking to see her granddaughter hooked up to so many tubes and looking so limp, like a Raggedy Ann doll. But even as she worried about Katie, she felt in some way guilty. So many of the children at Sloan-Kettering had cancer and were dying; their futures weren't all as hopeful as Katie's, who was being reborn.

At midmorning, Steve carried his son to the operating room. Christopher was flailing and grabbing on to Steve's hair. His belly was shaking from crying. Steve saw what looked to be about ten people waiting in scrubs.

It was Steve's first experience in an operating room, and it struck him that it looked just like the movies, down to the oversize white clock mounted on the wall. Steve held Christopher up to his shoulder as instructed, and he could smell the chemicals as a doctor put a mask over Christopher's nose and mouth to administer anesthesia. Steve held his breath because the smell was so bad. Looking at Christopher made him think of someone suffocating. Christopher's eyes rolled back in his head. After Christopher went limp, Steve set him on the operating table, kissed him, and left the room. He fought the eerie, uneasy feeling that came from leaving his son on a table, unconscious.

Steve donned a yellow gown, mask, and latex gloves and joined Stacy in Katie's room. Stacy's parents went out to get breakfast while Steve and Stacy entertained Katie for ninety minutes and waited to hear about Christopher. Stacy had dressed Katie in a pink T-shirt that said *I love Bubba*. Steve and Stacy had bought it on a trip to Manhattan, at the Bubba Gump Shrimp Company restaurant in Times Square. They thought it would be a perfect shirt for the day on which Christopher gave his sister a chance to be cured.

Wondering what was happening, Steve ventured to the recovery room despite the fact that the nurses hadn't called for him yet. As he entered, the nurses waved him over; they had just called Katie's room to tell him to come. The whole operation had been standard procedure, they told him. Once Christopher was out, the doctors had an easier time getting an IV in him and didn't need to go through the more dangerous leg vein. They took bone marrow from both of Christopher's hips, as planned.

Christopher's eyes were closed, but he was restlessly kicking his arms and legs. Steve picked him up and whispered into his ear, and Christopher immediately settled down and slept for two hours in his father's arms.

Stacy left Katie with her grandmother and came to see Christopher as well. Steve was holding Christopher and sitting against a window overlooking the buildings on First Avenue. A little blue tube blew oxygen onto Christopher's face. A bandage covered the spot where doctors had put the IV into Christopher's foot. He was wrapped in blankets.

————

At noon, Dr. Nancy Kernan walked into Katie's room with a blood bag filled with Christopher's marrow. Stacy was amazed it had arrived so quickly. The doctor hooked it to the Bubble Buddy attached to Katie's central line. The transplant was very similar to a blood transfusion in how it was administered: the marrow would drip into Katie over the span of four hours. She wouldn't feel a thing. As the marrow dripped, Katie watched *The Little Mermaid* on TV. She seemed entirely oblivious that anything was out of the ordinary.

Christopher's recovery went smoothly. When he woke at about one o'clock, he groggily sucked down a bottle of milk. Then he smiled. He was officially discharged about three. Steve took him to play in the Sloan-Kettering playroom, and Christopher toddled around, pushing a toy car. He didn't seem to be in any significant pain and would go home that day with a large bandage over puncture holes in his hips, just above his buttocks.

Stacy visited her son in the play area, and while she was there with Steve, Dr. Kernan came in. It seemed to Stacy as though the doctor, who usually had a poker face, was almost skipping. She sat down on a tiny chair meant for a toddler and told Steve and Stacy that she'd received the lab results back on the marrow they withdrew from Christopher and that the counts of stem cells they received were far better than they had anticipated. They had hoped for a CD 34 count of 5 million per kilo; Christopher's marrow had 19 million per kilo, more than three times the minimum necessary, Kernan told them. Steve and Stacy didn't understand all the medical jargon, but they understood Kernan's jubilant demeanor. The more stem cells, the higher the likelihood of the marrow engrafting in Katie, she told them. "He did a great job," she said.

Christopher seemed so normal—aside from his foot bothering him where the IV was inserted—that Stacy and Steve decided they could both stay with Katie, and they sent Christopher home to Long Island with Stacy's parents. They were relieved not to have to worry about Christopher anymore.

By dinnertime, the transplant was finished. Katie ate corn puffs cereal for dinner. She wanted a bagel but couldn't eat it because her mouth sores made it too painful. Stacy and Steve weren't surprised that Katie was still pretty normal, because doctors had explained that she would probably respond as she did on blood transfusion days and then have less energy in the coming weeks as her body fought to heal. Katie played for a while, pretending to wash down the walls of her room with bleach. She finally fell asleep at ten o'clock.

29

"Her Body Is Healing"

For months, Stacy had been wearing a red rubber LiveStrong-style Diamond Blackfan anemia bracelet. She never took it off. For the few days before the bone marrow transplant, it kept getting pulled off as she changed in and out of latex gloves, and she had to keep sliding it back on. The morning after Day Zero, she noticed that it was gone, and she asked Steve if he had seen it. "I saw it yesterday," he said, meaning he'd seen it on Stacy's wrist.

I lost it on transplant day, Stacy thought. It seemed an omen— Diamond Blackfan anemia, gone. Just like that.

The Trebings moved into the third phase of the transplant process: the post-transplant recovery at the hospital, which would likely last four weeks. Katie was not herself. Steve played Pretty Pretty Princess with her four times—usually she loved spinning the dial and racing to be the first to collect the princess ring and necklace and win the game. But Katie was listless. She just wanted to stay in bed watching *Tarzan*. She ate only half a Snickers bar and drank a Yoo-hoo. Confined in room 935, Stacy and Steve just sat. To Steve, every hour seemed three hours long.

But despite the boredom, Stacy felt optimistic, so lucky that things had gone so smoothly on the day of the transplant. She could do this hospital stay for another month, she thought. Boredom she could handle. As long as Katie was comfortable and didn't get sick. *This was a very, very, very good decision,* she told herself.

Stacy's sister Lisa called and mentioned Calvin. Everyone had been so effusive over Christopher the previous night, after the transplant. Now that they didn't have to worry about him being exposed to germs, family members could come visit, and everyone was making a big deal over how great Christopher did, how he saved his sister, Lisa said. Lisa noticed that Calvin seemed gloomy and took him aside to ask what was the matter. "I miss Mommy," he said. So Stacy asked her friends and family to pay special attention to Calvin if they visited the house in Nesconset and make a big fuss over him too.

Of the three Trebing children, Calvin, being the oldest, was the one that would remember the bone marrow ordeal most clearly, Stacy felt. She worried he would feel left out, not special. But Stacy knew she and Steve would repeatedly remind him that while Christopher had contributed his physical gift, Calvin had made other kinds of contributions. He was Katie's playmate and often entertained her and unknowingly gave her emotional support. He had made her a sign that hung in her hospital room that said, *Dear Katie, I hop yor feling Batr. I cant wat intil Yor bak becoos I hav nowon Two play with.*

Calvin was bright and energetic, and he had done so well in his private preschool that Stacy had worried he would be bored in public school. In the end, though, Calvin's transition into kindergarten had been difficult for him for other reasons. His kindergarten year had coincided with all the stressful months leading up to Katie's transplant, with Stacy and Steve spending so much time with Katie in the hospital. At the time, Katie's enormous medical needs had made it difficult for Stacy to handle any bumps in the road for Calvin. When Stacy received calls from Calvin's teacher reporting that he had been acting up in class, distracting the other children, she sobbed with guilt. She knew Calvin was acting out for attention, and she vowed to make it up to him when Katie was well.

At the Trebing household, Christopher was crawling around in his diaper, a bandage across his hips to protect the incision sites.

Pam and Cal Olsen were giving him Tylenol for any pain. Calvin got vitamins and fluoride. Even Hobbes, the dog, needed medicine. "I'm just hoping Christopher doesn't bark, because if he does, I made a mistake, and we have one serious problem," Pam joked.

"Twenty-four hours after giving bone marrow, look at him," an incredulous Pam said. Christopher was toddling around with his bottle, climbing with Calvin onto the treadmill. "Watch his back," Pam warned Calvin. Pam had given Christopher mashed potatoes for dinner as well as a steak bone that still had some meat on it for him to gnaw on. "A steak dinner for the king," she joked.

During the second week of waiting for Katie's blood cell counts to show that her body had accepted Christopher's marrow and begun making its own red blood cells, Steve left Stacy and Katie at Memorial Sloan-Kettering and went back to work for the first time since the transplant. He and his colleagues joked that *June* was a four-letter word for them—so much of their work putting up tents for weddings and graduations happened during that month. It was the worst possible time for Katie to be hospitalized.

That left Stacy handling the bulk of the time with Katie in the hospital. For the first two weeks after transplant, Stacy had one goal: keep Katie from getting any cold, fever, or infection before her immune system grew strong enough to handle an assault.

Caring for Katie was getting more tedious. Her hair was falling out, right on schedule, a few weeks after chemotherapy. Her head was now patchy, and the back was fuzzy because her hair got tugged out by the pressure of her head against the pillow. What bothered Katie the most was when hair fell in her food or on her toys. "Get it out of my Lucky Charms!" Katie would shout when eating breakfast.

Stacy posted pictures of Katie periodically on her CaringBridge Web site page, and Stacy's sister Lisa called to tell Stacy she should take down the most recent pictures. "She looks like death is on her doorstep. You're giving me a heart attack," Lisa said. Instead of upsetting Stacy, this made her laugh. "What did you expect her to look like? She's had chemotherapy. She's having a bone marrow transplant," Stacy reminded Lisa. The pictures of Katie dressing up in a tiara and makeup, with only tufts of hair left on her head, stayed put.

Katie did crafts much of each day, sitting in her bed. She made Popsicle-stick puppets with feathers and googly eyes. She made a princess crown and sparkle pictures. Once in a while, Katie reported matter-of-factly on how she was feeling. "I'm itching," she'd say. Or "My head hurts."

Some hours she was herself—calm and sweet, even in such a confined room. Then suddenly she would yell at Stacy. It was impossible for Stacy to predict what would set her off. Once Stacy answered the phone in her room by saying, "Katie's castle." "No!" Katie screamed. "Just 'Katie's room'!" Another time she yelled while Stacy was talking to a visitor to the room, "I don't like when Mommy talks to someone else! I hate you!" There was only so much "I hate you" Stacy could take. Once in a while, she cracked. Her eyes would tear and she would step outside the room for a moment. Fortunately, she knew that in a few minutes, Katie would be hugging her and telling her how much she loved her.

Stacy didn't know how much to discipline Katie; she didn't know if she was acting out because she was tired of being in the hospital or cranky because of the medicine or spoiled by the presents friends and family kept sending her and the undivided attention of whichever parent was by her bedside. Stacy decided it was okay if Katie had verbal outbursts—her rage making her face all red and crinkled—but that she'd draw the line if Katie smacked her or Steve or someone else.

Once, a priest made the rounds and stopped at Katie's door to bless her.

"Go away! Father, go away!" Katie yelled.

"Be nice, Katie," Stacy admonished. "Say, 'Have a nice day, Father.'"

The priest just smiled and lifted his right hand to bless Katie from the doorway. "It's a lot to get through," he said to Stacy with compassion.

One of Stacy's favorite parts of the long days was when Katie had to go to the bathroom. Because Stacy had to wear gloves and a mask, she never got to touch her daughter skin to skin. But when she picked Katie up to carry her into the bathroom, Katie put her head on Stacy's shoulder, and the skin on Stacy's neck touched the skin on Katie's face.

Every morning, as soon as she woke up, Stacy checked with the nurses to see what Katie's most recent blood tests showed. On the morning of June 8—two weeks post-transplant—Stacy woke up fully expecting Katie's bone marrow transplant to be kicking in. After all, Christopher had given such a good marrow sample, and Katie had been eating on her own, getting back some energy, making it through whole days without napping. So she was stunned when the nurses told her there was no evidence yet that Christopher's marrow had begun to take hold.

For a moment, Stacy felt like a fearful flier on an airplane. Katie still having no response at Day Fourteen was turbulence—the thought leaped into Stacy's mind that Katie wouldn't make it. Stacy so wished Katie's counts had come up before Stacy had had a chance to consider that they might not. She consoled herself with the knowledge that it had taken three weeks for Pete and Jen's son Jack's counts to return, and he was now doing great.

Then Stacy got more disappointing news. Steve, who had been out installing tents in the rain the day before, woke up with a runny nose. He was supposed to come to the hospital today for his shift, to let Stacy go home and see her boys. But now he'd be banished from Katie's world until all his symptoms disappeared. He also had to wait for a culture to come back so they'd know whether he had any infection, and that meant at least another five days of twenty-four/seven at the hospital for Stacy. That would make a total of ten days in a row for her.

The light at the end of my tunnel just went out, she thought.

Finally, after two more days that seemed like an eternity, Katie's blood tests indicated that Christopher's bone marrow was taking hold. Now that activity was brewing—now that Katie was beginning to make her own red blood cells—Stacy's mood shifted dramatically. Even though she was exhausted, she felt as though she could run a marathon. She started anticipating when they might go home. Stacy was counting the days—they'd already been in the hospital for nearly a month. She was hoping that they could go home in ten more days.

Now that Katie's immunity would also begin strengthening, though slowly, Stacy felt better about having a few select visitors. Her mom came to see Katie, donning the required gloves, mask, and yellow gown. She carried a little purple shopping bag with white tissue paper sticking out. It was a tapestry she'd embroidered herself to hang in Katie's hospital room. *Now I lay me down to sleep, I pray the Lord my soul to keep. May angels watch me through the night and wake me with the morning light,* it read. Pam had to look endlessly to find that wording. All of the other patterns had the traditional verse: *If I should die before I wake, I pray the Lord my soul to take.*

"What's new in your world?" Pam asked her granddaughter.

Katie, now completely bald, chatted happily. She pointed out the paper chain taped to the ceiling. "When I get to the brown one, I get to go home," she said. She offered Nana one of the chocolates she'd gotten from the candy cart. "It makes God happy when you share with everyone," Katie said.

But moments later, her mood swung and she yelled at Nana. "Stop copying me!" Katie yelled at Pam. "She's doing this," she said to Stacy, and Katie made a grimacing smile.

It was hard for Stacy and Pam to stifle laughter—there was no way Katie could tell what her Nana's smile looked like, because Pam was wearing a mask.

"But she has a mask on," Stacy pointed out to Katie.

"I see through it," Katie retorted.

"What am I doing now?" Nana asked.

Katie thought for a minute.

"You're eating Cheez Doodles!" she yelled.

Again, it was hard for Pam not to laugh.

At lunchtime, four doctors walked into the room, suited up with fresh gloves, masks, and gowns. They approached Katie, who was looking at a sticker book and eating dry Cheerios from a white plastic bowl, dipping them one by one into her Styrofoam milk cup as if they were cookies.

"Which picture do you like best?" Dr. Trudy Small asked Katie.

Katie pointed to the cat on the sticker-book cover.

"I like the puppy," Dr. Small said.

Katie's hemoglobin count, which indicated the level of red blood cells, was 10.9, closing in on a child's normal range of 12 to 16, Dr. Small told Stacy. Her retic count, a measure of young red blood cell production, was 1.2 percent, higher than it had ever been in her life and in the normal range. For the first time, Katie was making her own red blood cells. They were forming and growing until fully mature. Katie was still on track to go home in a week. Stacy could not believe that her child might never have to have a blood transfusion or use a Desferal pump again. It was a gift Stacy promised herself she would never take for granted.

"She's sleeping a lot," Stacy told Dr. Small. "Last night her whole body was aching. Her back hurt and her hands hurt."

"Her body is healing, and it's exhausting," Dr. Small said with compassion. She suggested hot packs to soothe Katie's back.

The doctors moved on to the next patient they had to see.

"Do you know what the reticulocyte counts are?" Stacy said to her mom, excited. "They're the precursors to the red blood cells, which is what they've always looked for. So when Katie was getting steroids, they kept checking her reticulocyte counts to see if anything was happening. Now she has them, because she has Bubba."

30

"Why Are You Taking the Lights Down?"

The healing progressed quickly during Katie's last week in Sloan-Kettering. Katie was allowed to leave her room for the first time. Stacy put a mask and gloves on her, and she cut down a yellow gown so Katie could walk without tripping. Katie ventured into the hallway and ran after the clowns as they visited room to room. It seemed everything Stacy and Steve had been hoping and praying for was happening.

Stacy started to make a list of the germ-fighting protocol everyone would have to follow when Katie got home, because it could take up to a year for Katie's immune system to be normal. *Come in and out only the garage entrance,* Stacy wrote. *Take shoes off in the mudroom and use hand sanitizer there before entering the house. Send Hobbes the Saint Bernard to Steve's parents' house. Clean carpet. Buy Katie a new mattress.*

In Nesconset, Stacy's sister Lisa enlisted her mom, her niece, and several others to clean the Trebing house, wiping down the walls with disinfectant. Lisa was nervous about Katie's transition home—she would be housebound for months because her immune system would still be weak. So many things could still go wrong.

Lisa worried about Katie coming home to two active brothers bringing in germs. In fact, Steve's parents had just left the house with Calvin and Christopher, taking them to Fire Island until they could be declared healthy enough to come home and see Katie. Both of them had colds.

The cleaning team met at seven thirty that evening at Steve and Stacy's. They posted an octagonal red stop sign on the front door and a note directing people to the garage entrance. At the garage entrance, they hung another stop sign and put a handwritten notice underneath that said, *Please Take Off Shoes. Wash Hands. No Colds, Please.* A picture of a skull and crossbones emphasized the warning.

"What do we want to do with this dining room?" Pam Olsen asked. She was armed with Windex and Lysol wipes.

"Why do I have to make all the executive decisions?" Lisa jokingly griped. "I guess wipe down stuff. The door, the chairs." On the table was a lime green loose-leaf notebook. Inside was the paperback book *Me and My Marrow*. Stacy had given a copy to each of her sisters and to her mom as well.

There was a knock at the garage door. It was Kelsey Gilmartin, a sixteen-year-old neighbor. She'd come to make a welcome-home banner for Katie. Lisa had bought paper and purple paint, Katie's favorite color. She'd also bought red, white, and blue windmills to stick on the front lawn. She unwrapped a glass wind chime. "I thought this would be nice too. She can't go out too much, so she can hear the wind chimes."

Inside the house, the older generation of women was getting punch-drunk. Pam was in the bathroom, sitting on the toilet seat as she wiped down the molding. Helen Conklin, Pam's cousin, walked into the bathroom. "Is this done?" Helen asked.

"I'm in here. Can't I have any privacy? Can't you see I'm sitting?" Pam deadpanned. Lisa walked in from the garage, and Pam and Helen faked sneezing and coughing.

"Meanwhile, my house hasn't been vacuumed all week," Lisa grumbled, not appreciating their humor. She reached to open a kitchen cabinet.

"Don't touch the knobs!" Helen said.

"I'm looking for the garbage bags," Lisa said.

"Use a wipe!" Helen said. "You're supposed to do this"—she held the knob with a wipe and opened the cabinet.

"Look. I'm not going to close the cabinet with my hand. I'll close it with my foot," Lisa said.

"That's worse!" Helen said.

Lisa barely resisted rolling her eyes.

On Wednesday, June 21, 2006—thirty-seven days after Katie checked into Memorial Sloan-Kettering for her bone marrow transplant—Stacy woke and pulled down the string of lights she had put up that first day.

"Why are you taking the lights down?" Katie asked.

"Because we're going home. We're not sleeping here tonight," Stacy said.

"I have to eat my macaroni and cheese and then I can go home," Katie said. She was hiding marbles under plastic medicine cups on her tray.

Steve was also in Manhattan, across the city, sweating at Tavern on the Green on the Upper West Side, installing a tent with a dozen of his guys. They had one day to erect an enormous tent with white peaks, a runway, air-conditioning. It was his company's busiest week of the year; he had five other major jobs going on simultaneously. Stacy's mom, Stacy's sister Leslie, and Stacy's niece Sammy would drive into the city to pick Stacy and Katie up and bring them home.

At noon, the phone rang in Katie's room. It was Sammy. The women were parking at a garage on East Seventieth Street. "Sounds good," Stacy said. "Have you got the cookies?" Stacy and Steve were leaving two big platters of bakery cookies, one for the nursing staff and one in the family common area. "Take your time. They still have to pull her central line out and then she has to sit for an hour."

Stacy hung up. "That was your cousin Sammy," she said to Katie. "She's on her way."

"Then we're going home?" Katie asked hopefully.

"They've got to take your line out first." Most children who have had bone marrow transplants went home with their central lines still in. But Stacy had pleaded with the doctors to take Katie's out. It was a potential source of infection, and if Katie got a fever she would have to come back to Sloan-Kettering immediately because it could indicate a dangerous infection in the central line. The doctors liked to leave the lines in because the patients would continue to need blood tested when they came back for outpatient visits, and taking blood through the central line didn't upset children like getting stuck with a needle did. But Katie had been receiving IV needles all her life, and Stacy thought this would not be an issue. So the doctors agreed.

The entourage arrived. Pam Olsen took out a paper robe and looked at Sammy. "What color do you want? Yellow or yellow?" she joked.

"Yellow," Sammy answered.

"What's that big red thing for?" Katie asked, pointing to an empty suitcase.

"That's for your stuff to go in," Aunt Leslie said.

Stacy and Leslie took down a plastic blow-up palm tree that Leslie had sent as a gift weeks earlier; it had been decorating the room. "I wanted to give it to someone who's staying here, but Katie wants to take it home," Stacy told Leslie.

"What are you going to do with it?" Leslie asked Katie.

"I don't know," Katie said.

Stacy got up on a chair and reached up to take down Katie's last construction paper loop, still taped, all alone, to the ceiling.

At two fifteen, a doctor came in to take out Katie's central line, disconnecting her from the IV stand for the first time in thirty-seven days. He snipped what he thought were all the sutures and tried to tug the line out. Katie screamed and kicked her feet. Pam and Leslie left the room, uncomfortable watching Katie crying in pain. "Maybe there's another suture," the doctor said, and sure enough there was, crusted over with old blood. He cut that one. Katie was still kicking and screaming.

"Congratulations, you're free," the nurse on duty said as she wheeled the disconnected Bubble Buddy away.

"Boy, there's a lot of room in here without Bubble Buddy," Stacy said. She started to change Katie into the clothes she would wear home. "Mommy, put gloves on," Katie said. Stacy was concerned about how worried they had made Katie about germs. Yesterday, when Katie had to have some final ultrasounds, she was nervous about sitting in the hospital waiting area. She wanted to go back to the room, saying, "I'm going to get germs."

"I washed my hands. I washed them very good," Stacy assured her.

By three thirty, Katie had had it. When the nurse came back, Katie yelled, "I want to go home!" Everyone laughed.

The nurse had paperwork for Stacy to sign and medications for her to take home. She put Katie in a wheelchair to leave the hospital. Katie wore a mask and latex gloves that were too big for her and that flopped off the ends of her fingers. As Stacy pushed Katie to the elevator, Katie passed by the priest who had visited her several times during her transplant stay and whom she had more than once kicked out of her room.

"Katie, you're going home," the priest said. "God bless you."

By four o'clock, Aunt Leslie was maneuvering the minivan through the Manhattan traffic. Katie watched *Barbie Fairytopia* and ate a banana. Stacy felt a jolt of panic: Katie wasn't in a controlled environment anymore. Even though they had had Leslie's car cleaned and washed Katie's car seat, Stacy still worried. Katie fell asleep during the movie and woke up right around the block from home.

"We're almost home, Katie," Sammy said, excitement in her voice. "We're right down the block."

"That way!" Katie directed Aunt Leslie.

"How'd you get so smart?" Stacy asked.

"I got lots of hugs," Katie said. Stacy always told her children that hugs made them smarter.

When they pulled in the driveway, Katie tried to yank off her seat belt. She wanted to see the pinwheels on the lawn, but she wasn't allowed to step on the grass, so Stacy carried her to the front door. They went inside and Stacy set Katie down. Katie dashed into the kitchen. "Where's Cal? Where's Christopher? Where's Daddy?" she said. "Where's all the people?" Stacy told Katie that her brothers were on Fire Island because they had colds and that her dad would be home later.

Leslie's husband, Joe, walked over from the landscaping nursery and stood at the screen door to the kitchen. He was afraid to come in, fearful that he would bring in germs that could hurt Katie. Instead he peered through the opening like the Scarecrow in *The Wizard of Oz* when Dorothy says, "There's no place like home."

"Nice to see you home, honey," Uncle Joe said to Katie.

Within a few days, Calvin and Christopher were well enough to come back.

At first, Stacy had Katie wear a surgical mask around her brothers for fear she could still catch some germs from the boys. Steve's parents drove Calvin and Christopher home; when Stacy's parents saw the car coming down the street, they walked over to see the reunion.

It wasn't exactly the reunion Stacy had imagined.

As soon as Christopher saw Katie—bald and wearing a mask—he screamed. Stacy thought Christopher didn't realize he was looking at his sister. And Christopher's reaction to Stacy was nonplussed. Stacy felt like he was mad at her for leaving him for so long and had decided he didn't care whether she was there or not.

Calvin, on the other hand, was unfazed. "She's not that bald," he said, alluding to the fuzz on Katie's head.

"I love you," Katie said to Calvin and Christopher. "I love my brothers."

Stacy took off Katie's mask for a minute and Christopher stopped crying. Katie hugged him. She hugged Calvin. "I love you," she said again and again, even though Christopher was still treating her like a stranger.

Calvin and Katie climbed on the couch with Stacy and Christopher, and Stacy started to cry. It felt so good, after a month and a half, to hold all three of her children together.

31

"Back Up and Bling-Bling"

Stacy was alarmed when she noticed a rash traveling up Katie's belly and back a few days after they'd arrived home. She knew it must have something to do with Katie's body reacting to the new bone marrow. She called Sloan-Kettering, and they wanted to see it. Immediately. She called Steve, who had gone to work for the day, and he came home so he could go with them. Stacy packed an overnight bag just in case. But once the doctors saw the rash, they weren't overly concerned. Katie had to come in the next day for a scheduled follow-up visit anyway, so the doctors would check it again then.

When they got back home to Nesconset, Stacy took advantage of Steve's being home to go over to a neighbor's. Calvin was at his cousin's watching a movie; Steve was alone with Christopher and Katie. Katie was lying without a mask on Steve's lap, watching TV in the living room, just like she used to before she went into the hospital. Christopher stood in the living room, watching them oddly.

Steve thought that was when Christopher finally realized Katie was Katie. Suddenly, he ran over and grabbed Katie's face. He pulled her head toward him and started kissing her, right on the lips. Steve was startled and somewhat alarmed, because the kids weren't supposed to do anything that might exchange germs. Steve tried to separate them, but Katie was giggling. "Oh, he loves me," she said.

The Trebings had taught Christopher, who wasn't talking yet, the sign-language sign for *more*. He used it when he wanted more food or another bottle. He started making the *more* sign to Steve. Steve gave in. "Katie, he wants more," Steve said. And to Christopher: "Just don't kiss her on the lips." Christopher kissed his sister ten times on the nose.

As Stacy was putting Katie to bed, Katie told her the story. "When I came home from the hopital," she said, leaving out the *s,* "Christopher was scared because I had no hair. He realized it was me, and now he's happy."

"Are you happy?" Stacy asked her daughter.

"I'm so happy," Katie replied.

Subsequent trips to Memorial Sloan-Kettering provided a diagnosis of Katie's rash: mild graft-versus-host disease. Christopher's marrow was rattling Katie's body, causing angry red bumps. Katie would need oral steroids for four to six months to battle it. But because steroids suppressed the immune system, they would delay her return to everyday life.

The Trebings already knew they were in for a long haul at home—doctors had warned that post-transplant recovery lasted up to a year. Patients initially returned to Sloan-Kettering three times a week; this was reduced to once a week as patients improved. While Day One Hundred after transplant usually was a milestone in the process, it was far from the end. Which meant the Trebings still lived connected to the hospital. Stacy rose at five thirty on the summer days she had to drive Katie to checkups. Katie's blood had to be taken at a certain interval between medications, so Stacy had to arrive at eight. The drive could take up to two hours each way, depending on traffic conditions.

Even inside the house, the Trebings continued to fear germs. Purell hand sanitizer bottles were visible on every room's windowsill, like holiday candles. Stacy couldn't order takeout, which carried the threat of germs, so when she got home from the hospital, she still had to cook dinner. Preparing Katie's food was tedious—

Stacy avoided cutting through fruit when peeling it, for instance, so the knife wouldn't contaminate the inside.

On top of this, Katie took eight medicines, some multiple times daily. Tacrolimus to fight graft-versus-host disease. Prednisone—the steroid—to do the same. Acyclovir to prevent viruses. Prevacid to protect her stomach from the steroids. Fluconazole to prevent fungus. And so on. She took some medications at 9:00 a.m., some at 10:00, others at noon, and still others at 5:00 p.m. Stacy had to keep all that straight and had to coax Katie into swallowing them. Steve took the night shift, getting up for the 1:00 a.m. dose.

Katie couldn't leave the house. She used paper towels, not hand towels that could harbor germs. She had her own bathroom no one else used. Any time a family member came inside, shoes had to be removed in the mudroom and hands sanitized. The Trebings called cleaning their hands bling-blinging because they had bought an automated unit that chimed as it dispensed sanitizer. As Calvin came in from playing, Stacy could hear whether he'd cleaned his hands. "Back up and bling-bling," she'd yell from the kitchen.

Stacy was in a perpetual state of fatigue. Taking care of three children, two under age five, would have been exhausting enough. But keeping Katie entertained indoors, waking up at night to give Christopher a bottle, and rising at five thirty to drive Katie into Manhattan made rest little more than a fantasy. Steve was also spent; he was working sunup to sundown supervising the installation of tents for weddings and parties, trying to recoup some of the money the business had lost during the stretch when he was unable to work due to Katie's hospitalization.

On the way home from the hospital one day, Stacy thought about a time when she was pregnant with Christopher and Katie was in preschool. After Katie's class, the moms would take the kids to a nearby playground. One day, a mother with three kids was teasing Stacy, warning her that when she had her third child and tried to bring all three to the playground at once, it would be hellish. "Each one will be running in a different direction and you'll have to chase them all," she said. That's what Stacy daydreamed about on her drive home—bringing her three healthy children to the playground and not worrying if they got dirty or sweaty or came away teeming with germs. Then they could all pile in the car and get ice cream, no one fretting about Katie being served outside the cocoon of their house.

Fortunately, there were moments when Stacy saw a rainbow. For instance, she always shopped at the same supermarket and frequently chatted with the same cashier. One week, while Stacy was checking out, the cashier asked how Katie was doing. The woman behind Stacy had the same Gap shirt on as Stacy did and also had a daughter named Katie, so they started to chat as well. Nothing unusual about that.

Stacy was packing the car when the woman ran up to her. She had asked the cashier what the problem was with Katie. "I had a bone marrow transplant when I was eighteen," the woman told Stacy excitedly. Dr. Boulad had been her doctor too. "He came to my wedding," she said. "He saved my life." Stacy couldn't linger and talk for as long as she wanted; Calvin and Christopher were waiting in the car, frozen food was melting. But the woman did tell Stacy that her brother had been her donor too, and that she now had two adopted children from China. Stacy felt her eyes well up with tears; Katie's future was standing right before her. This woman was living proof of Stacy's dream of Katie growing up healthy and having a family. Before they parted, the two women hugged.

In mid-July, doctors gave Katie permission to go swimming in her grandmother's pool next door, as long as she wore a long-sleeved shirt and a hat to protect her from the sun, and a mask to protect her from germs. The whole family walked over for a dip. Stacy and Steve used a white bedsheet to construct a covering across the pool steps to shade Katie, but she refused to be confined. She stepped into a lavender tube. "Watch this!" she yelled and jumped in. Cal did a flying eagle off the diving board.

"I'm going to get dizzy," Katie said gleefully, and she kicked her legs to twirl herself around in her float. "Katie, you're not supposed to do that," Calvin reprimanded his sister. "You can get really dizzy, and you can drown in the water."

Nana and Pop were sitting under a nearby tree, and Pam was trying to entice Christopher into the shade by offering him a soccer ball. He was more interested in dancing to a CD of Calvin's twenty favorite songs. "He cracks me up, that guy," Calvin said of his grandson Christopher. "Another couple of years and the other two won't stand a chance."

"We nicknamed him Schwarzenegger," Pam said, because Christopher seemed to have such a solid build.

Pam was not as nervous about Katie anymore. Katie's visits to Sloan-Kettering had been reduced to once a week, every Monday. Watching her granddaughter splashing in the pool, Pam thought it seemed like Katie would, indeed, soon return to normal.

During the third week of August, eighty-eight days after Katie had received Christopher's bone marrow, a blood test at Sloan-Kettering showed Katie's body was still making its own new red blood cells. But her T cells, the soldiers for fighting infection, were still far too low for Katie to return to normal activity, just as doctors had expected would be the case at this point.

When they were ready to leave the hospital, Katie made a request. "I want to go say good-bye to Dr. Boulad," she told Stacy. "I want to hug him and I want to kiss him and tell him I love him." They found Boulad in his ninth-floor office. "Thank you for making me better," Katie said, as Boulad, with Katie on his lap, spun in his desk chair. Stacy watched with a lump in her throat. Boulad had a lump in his as well.

Day One Hundred came on Saturday, September 2, two years and one day after Stacy learned she was pregnant with Christopher. It was the day the Trebings had believed would mark a watershed— the acceptance of Christopher's bone marrow and the vanquishing of Katie's DBA. Stacy still felt Day One Hundred was some sort of benchmark. Stacy and Steve would be going to a wedding that night, and Stacy had bought a new black halter dress so she could celebrate with Steve, even though Katie had yet to be given the all-clear to return to all normal activities.

By then, Katie was stronger, doing more outdoor things—she was allowed to ride a bike on the street in front of the house, for instance—but she had to wear a mask and gloves. Still, she was making plans for the future. "When I get all better, I'm going to the beach and I'm going to bring everyone," Katie said one night. And "When I get better, I'm going to Chuck E. Cheese."

On Halloween, Sloan-Kettering threw its annual costume party, and Katie was permitted back into the outpatient children's playroom at the hospital for the first time. The playroom had been transformed. Black cats arched their backs on the wall, and dozens of Mylar balloons shaped like white ghosts with wide smiles, bats with purple neon stripes, and creepy spiders hung from the ceiling. Katie wore a fairy princess costume with wings. She also had to wear her surgical mask.

"You look great!" "You look wonderful!" Staff members dressed as cowgirls and Native American princesses gloated over Katie. Dr. Nancy Kernan, the doctor who did Christopher's marrow extraction and Katie's transplant, was there as a witch. She hugged Katie, then phoned her secretary. "I just ran into a princess who could benefit from one of my wands that light up," she said. One was delivered to Katie.

A magician named Magic Juan entertained. "Say 'poof,'" he instructed. "Poof!" Katie and the other children yelled. "Don't say poop! Who said poop?" Magic Juan cried, indignant. Katie's eyes crinkled, evidence of her smile behind the mask.

In December, Katie took over questioning Boulad at a routine appointment. "When can my dog come home?" she demanded.

Boulad looked at Katie's latest blood test results in an exaggerated way, then smiled. "She can come now."

Katie leaped out of the chair and hugged him.

"What else do you want?" Boulad asked her.

"Can I go back to school?"

"Yes," he said.

Katie hugged him again.

"What else?"

It was like Boulad had morphed into Santa and Katie's requests came tripping out. "Can I eat grapes? Can I have strawberries?" Both had been banned because they carried the risk of bacteria.

"As long as Mommy washes them well," Boulad granted.

Stacy wasn't about to be left out of all the hugging, and she embraced Boulad as well. *How do I say thank you to this man who has guided my child to victory?* she thought.

That afternoon, Stacy picked up Hobbes from her in-laws' house, where the Saint Bernard had been for more than six months. Hobbes came home just in time for Katie's fourth birthday, on December 12. And the Trebings threw caution to the winds and took Katie to her preschool's holiday party.

The Trebings had their traditional Christmas Eve family party at their house. They invited Stacy's mom and dad and her sisters, Lisa and Leslie, and their families. Katie wore a giraffe-skin-patterned skirt and a pink fuzzy magenta shirt with a light pink dog on it. Her hair had still not fully grown in. Christopher wore a little suit, his bow tie askew.

Stacy's dad sneaked out, came back dressed as Santa, and dropped off a sack of gifts for the kids. Katie got the jewelry box she'd wanted.

"It's hard to transition from 'You can't do anything' to 'The dog can come home, you can go back to school, and you can eat whatever you want,'" said Steve as he stood by the fireplace. He was happy about the new edict, but it just seemed so surreal.

On New Year's Eve, as 2006 gave way to 2007, Stacy's prayer of the previous New Year's Eve was answered. Katie looked at Stacy and said, "Happy New Year, Mommy."

32

"It Goes So Fast"

"Step on in, my darling," said Miss Stephanie in early January when Stacy brought Katie back to preschool for the first time since her transplant. "Every day I've been waiting for you." Stephanie Shlachtman showed Katie the attendance sheet with Katie's name on it. "I can put a check now. That's so exciting to me."

Stacy reminded Miss Stephanie that any fruit Katie ate had to be washed well. "Katie, I put your Purell in your backpack," Stacy said to Katie as she joined the circle of children, putting down her Team Strawberry backpack with the cheerleader on it.

But two days later, Katie told Stacy she didn't want to go to school. At circle time, she explained, all the other kids already knew the alphabet. They already had their friends and didn't want to play with her; they stared at her still-patchy hair. "I want to stay home with you," Katie said.

Then Katie got strep throat. A few days later, an ear infection. Katie seemed extremely prone to illnesses, even though her immune system was fighting them. But the sicknesses meant added medication, and Stacy wanted to be done with all of that. *Is she ever going to be normal?* Stacy wondered. She had been naive, thinking the bone marrow transplant would turn off all Katie's problems as neatly as a light switch. Steve and Stacy pulled Katie back out of school.

But if it wasn't school getting Katie sick, it was her brothers.

Just as the Trebings were ready to leave for their long-awaited Make-A-Wish Foundation trip to Disney World in early February, Christopher got a rash. The Make-A-Wish Foundation fulfilled wishes of children with life-threatening diseases; most of them, including Katie, wanted to go to Orlando. Stacy took Christopher to the pediatrician—he had fifth disease. The pediatrician believed Katie also had it. The viral illness was common in young children and produced a signature red rash on the face, which could spread. Fifth disease was an ordinary childhood illness for a healthy child. But for an immunosuppressed child such as Katie, the virus could attack her new bone marrow.

Stacy called Boulad; he was busy with patients so she explained what was going on to his secretary. Stacy was at a Taco Bell drive-through when her cell phone rang. As soon as Stacy heard Boulad's voice, she knew it was going to be bad news.

"We have to talk about the fifth disease," Boulad said. It could attack Katie's bone marrow up to three weeks after exposure, and it could be life-threatening. He warned Stacy to bring Katie to Sloan-Kettering if anything at all seemed amiss.

"So you know what that means?" Boulad asked.

"That I have to be walking on eggshells for two weeks?" Stacy said.

"Yes. Do you know what else that means?"

"That we can't go to Disney?"

"Yes," Boulad said.

Stacy called the Make-A-Wish people and they rescheduled the family trip to April, the week after Easter. Everyone was disappointed.

The days passed without Katie getting worse. So on Monday, April 9, Katie packed her American Girl suitcase for Florida, the same one she'd rolled into Sloan-Kettering nearly a year ago. Her red blood cell counts were strong; the fifth disease threat was over; her immune system was stronger than it had been since the transplant. Her hair had grown in; it was still short, but it was full. The doctors were weaning Katie off of her drugs, though it would still take a few months until she was completely free of them.

"I need sunscreen," Katie said to Stacy as she packed.

"I've got that covered," Stacy said.

"We need diapers for Bubba," Katie said.

"I've got that covered too," Stacy said.

When Steve came home at four thirty, Christopher and Katie were watching a Disney vacation-planning video in the basement. Steve sat next to Katie on the couch; she was sandwiched between mom and dad. "You're my best mom and dad ever," Katie said.

"Thanks, Katie," said Steve.

Just days after they got home from the trip to Disney World, Stacy got the go-ahead to schedule Katie for a battery of testing that would enable her to move on to a different doctor at Sloan-Kettering, one who would see Katie just every six months through puberty to make sure she continued to thrive.

The final cost to cure Katie of her Diamond Blackfan anemia had topped $325,000. Of that amount, the Trebings' insurance company had paid approximately $164,000, covering Katie's liver biopsy and the thirty-seven-day stay at Memorial Sloan-Kettering Cancer Center. The insurance company also paid approximately $86,000 for outpatient services at the cancer center. Steve and Stacy Trebing paid $35,000 for the procedures that resulted in Christopher's birth, $5,000 to have Katie's ovary frozen, and $35,000 in doctor-visit and drug co-pays and other items such as expenses driving back and forth to Sloan-Kettering and installing an air-filter system in their home to remove germs and mold that could be dangerous to Katie. That $325,000 total doesn't include various doctors' fees at Sloan-Kettering as well as follow-up care at Stony Brook University Medical Center.

At Katie's ballet class in the third week of April, one of the other mothers asked Stacy about Katie's medical issues. Stacy was characteristically open about it, explaining to a group of mothers everything she and Steve had gone through as the group watched their daughters twirl and plié in the studio, dressed in pink tutus and bodysuits.

"She had Diamond Blackfan anemia," Stacy said. "She didn't make any red blood cells."

"Wow," said Tara Dickson, whose four-year-old daughter, Gianna, was dancing near Katie.

Stacy explained how Katie had had a bone marrow transplant last May, nearly a year ago, and how Christopher was selected from Stacy and Steve's embryos to be her donor.

"We went through IVF, two cycles, and we had him on the second cycle," Stacy explained.

"Part of the reason you had him was to help her, in a sense?" asked Dickson.

"Yes," Stacy said. "We were going to have a third child anyway."

"That's great," Dickson said.

"We froze her ovary," Stacy continued.

"Holy cow," Dickson said.

"Unbelievable," said another mother.

"She's got the best of modern science," Stacy said. "It's been some ride."

Stacy opened a candle shaped like the number 2, and Katie stuck it on the sheet cake.

"Bring Bubba!" Katie demanded. Christopher was in the Trebing backyard, jumping on the trampoline. "Bubba!"

A streak of boy ran through the screen door. He bounded onto the same chair with Katie, Calvin hovering behind them. Christopher blew out the candle, Katie kissed her little brother on the cheek, and he promptly stuck his finger into the green icing and then into his mouth.

It was May of 2007, Christopher's second-birthday party. This was the shindig the Trebings hadn't been able to have last year when Bubba turned one because they were just two weeks from checking into Memorial Sloan-Kettering for Katie's bone marrow transplant.

"I can't believe it. It goes so fast," Steve said, taking a break from grilling hamburgers and hot dogs to join dozens of family and friends in the singing of "Happy Birthday." "It seems like yesterday he was born, and now he's two. We kind of lost that first year. We couldn't have people over. This is his first birthday party."

"Bubba gets the first slice," bossed Katie. "He's the birthday boy."

Stacy handed Christopher a plate.

"Happy birthday to you!" Katie yelled.

The Trebing celebrations would continue all summer.

A few days later, Katie was a guest of honor at the annual black-tie Bone Marrow Foundation fund-raising dinner in Manhattan, which raised $800,000 to help families with medical costs. Cameras flashed in a cacophony of light as paparazzi shot Katie with the evening's co-host Meredith Vieira, the evening's entertainment Rihanna, and finally Sarah Jessica Parker.

A waitress passed by serving caviar hors d'oeuvres. "Got any chicken nuggets?" Stacy quipped. At dinner, Calvin, in a tuxedo, pulled a funny-shaped mushroom from his salad plate and held it up like a smelly sock. "Ew," he said, and Steve, also in a tux, shot him a warning look. At ten o'clock, Katie was asleep on Dad's lap.

In July, doctors took Katie off all medications. Boulad delivered the news: Katie's deadly Diamond Blackfan anemia had been conquered. Christopher's bone marrow did what it was supposed to do—it altered Katie's fate. Katie had her first appointment with Charles Sklar, the physician at Memorial Sloan-Kettering who monitored bone marrow transplant recipients long-term and would examine Katie periodically through puberty. Katie still had an increased risk of some cancerous tumors and would need to have occasional blood withdrawals done at her local hospital to remove previously accumulated iron from her liver.

During August, the Trebings vacationed at Steve's parents' Fire

Island house. All five Trebings headed to the ocean, on the same stretch of sand where, three years before, Stacy had told Steve that her hormone levels were low and it was possible that she might be miscarrying.

Where he'd kissed her belly and urged Bubba to hang on.

Steve swung Christopher through the waves, Katie darted through the surf shadowed by Hobbes, and Calvin skim-boarded along the shoreline.

In early September, in what seemed to Stacy like the final indication that life had returned to normal, Katie headed back to preschool. She was almost five. Stacy had made a construction paper chart that she hung on the refrigerator with pictures of chores Katie had to do before she left for school—brush her teeth, get dressed, pack her snack. Katie was up at seven, so excited she didn't go back to sleep even though her program didn't start until ten thirty.

"It's my special day," Katie proclaimed, all ready in a brown dress with pink polka dots, a lavender heart barrette holding back her now grown-in hair. "We're going to do painting, and play with Play-Doh."

"Let's check your backpack to make sure you have everything," Stacy said.

Katie sat on the kitchen floor. She stuck her head completely inside her backpack, pulling out first her lunch box and then her school folder. She poked her head in again, but saw she'd already taken out everything.

She looked up.

"That's the end of the story, folks," she announced.

ACKNOWLEDGMENTS

For those of you who believe there are no coincidences, I contribute this story to the body of supporting evidence. We have a counter at *Newsday*, where "The Match" project began, on which reporters and editors put books they don't need anymore. Two-thirds of the way through the project, I noticed a book called *Choosing Naia*. On the cover was a pregnant woman being embraced by her husband. The couple had to choose whether to have their baby, whom they knew would be born with Down syndrome. *Choosing Naia* seemed like the kind of book my series "The Match" might one day become. I took the book, and it sat on a corner of my desk through the remaining months of reporting and writing.

When the Trebing story ran in *Newsday*, many people suggested it be expanded. One was my great friend and colleague Letta Tayler. "You should contact my friend Mitchell Zuckoff for advice on how to get a book published," she said to me. "He wrote a book called *Choosing Naia* based on a series he did for the *Boston Globe*."

I was amazed by the coincidence (but of course, there are no coincidences), and I e-mailed Mitchell. He immediately called me. He offered excellent advice and passed my *Newsday* series on to his *Choosing Naia* publisher, Helene Atwan at Beacon Press in Boston. Thank you, Mitchell, so much. I hope this book has approached your superb level of storytelling.

Helene immediately believed in this project and has been its guiding light. From our first meeting at the Beacon Press offices in Boston in March of 2008, I believed in Helene just as much. I feel blessed that she became the editor of this book. I also salute members of the Beacon staff Robyn Day, Susan Lumenello, Tom Hallock, Pam MacColl, and Tracy Roe.

I am grateful to my many journalist friends who were generous with the names of their book agents, and I'm especially indebted to Brian Donavan, who shared Robert Guinsler of Sterling Lord Literistic with me. Robert has been a support and cheering section and gave me supreme confidence in the agreement I made.

I must thank my colleagues at *Newsday* who put their hearts into "The Match" as it was being reported, written, and published in the newspaper. Closest to the project were photographer Bill Davis and videographer John Paraskevas. Bill and I became—in the words of Stacy Trebing—like an old married couple. It was probably the eight-hour-plus road trip to meet the Zangrando family and the Johnsons in Ohio that cemented our comfort with each other. Bill captured the Trebings' emotions in ways that words could not. John was videographer extraordinaire, getting down on the ground to film a crawling Christopher and taping hours of family dinners and interviews with Stacy and Steve. Thanks also to Bill's wife, our colleague Liane Guenther, for her support.

Then there were the colleagues whom I've often referred to as the "swarm of bees." First among them was *Newsday* editor John Mancini, who came up with the brilliant title for the series, which is also the title of this book. Debbie Henley was the patron saint of the print version, and Debby Krenek worked past midnight many nights to get the Web site up and running smoothly. Publisher Tim Knight was an ardent supporter as well. Thanks to *Newsday* editors Genetta Adams, Margaret Corvini, Alex Martin, Barbara Schuler, and Phyllis Singer. I've saved the most important editor for last: Steve Wick. His insight and ability to edit narrative is astounding, and my respect for him is boundless. Reporters often wind up hating their editors by the end of their projects; I liked mine even better at the finale. Thanks go as well to Jeff Schamberry, Andrea Miller, Andrew Wong, Rod Eyer, Leema Thomas, Jonathan McCarthy, Arnold Miller, Joe Garraffo, Tony Jerome, and Barbara Teleha. My gratitude also to Mary Ann Skinner, who shepherded the company approval of this book.

Gail Deutsch and Farnaz Javid at ABC's *20/20* threw themselves into a television piece based on the series.

Dr. Jeffrey Lipton at Schneider Children's Hospital is a phenomenally dedicated doctor who was endlessly available to answer my countless questions through e-mail, over the phone, and in person. Dr. James Stelling of Reproductive Specialists of New York is another impressive physician and the reason I was able to tell this story, as he connected me with the Trebing family. My thanks go as well to Dr. Farid Boulad at Memorial Sloan-Kettering Cancer Center for his unwavering support.

No book can be written without the understanding of friends and family. Especially supportive have been Valerie Kellogg, Marjorie Robins, Denise Flaim, Amanda Barrett, Dave Marcus, Erica Marcus, Joe Haberstroh, Rebecca Alford, and Dolores and Denise Lupion. Thanks also to my colleagues and friends at Columbia University, especially Laura Muha and Sam Freedman, who were generous with their advice and encouragement. Thanks to Dan Fagin, who pointed me to the respected scientific competitions that led to "The Match" winning the National Association of Science Writers' Science in Society award. Cousin Robert Ziegler saved me from complete panic by magically restoring my laptop after Diet Dr Pepper spilled on the keyboard. Rosario "Charo" Sanchez and Eduardo Sanchez both pitched in to help me during the most stressful points in the publishing schedule.

Thanks to my first readers—Team Book—Linda Bold, Jeanine Debar, Karen Hinton, Tammy Rosenthal, Melissa Ryan, and Joan Weiner. They also happen to be among my best friends. My gratitude also to Amir Rosenthal, who lent me his legal mind.

I wish that my grandmother Bobbie were alive to read this; she always nudged me to write a book and would have loved to see it. Thanks to my sister, Karen Hinton, who always takes my neurotic phone calls, and her husband, Dave, who doesn't (usually) object to them, and to my late brother, Gene, who we wish had had a sibling match himself; he needed a kidney transplant, which he didn't live long enough to receive. Thanks also to my nieces and nephews, Bryan and Amanda Hinton and Russell and Tamara Whitehouse, and to my sister-in-law Elva Woodard.

Thank you to my mom and dad, Sandra and Donald Whitehouse, for both their nature and nurture. They gave me their superlative genes and an unparalleled upbringing. My mom made myriad trips to help me care for my son and accomplish travel needed for this project. I love you, Mom and Dad.

During this project, I met Greg Lupion. I have been blessed with many professional opportunities but not so many chances to have the family I'd always dreamed of. Greg has made that dream come true and filled my life with romantic happiness. We married as this book was going to press. I now live with my husband and his daughter, Miranda, whom I refer to as my bonus child, and my always treasured son, Tristan. Tristan, because of you, I understand viscerally why parents would go to any lengths to cure their children. I am so proud of what a great student, soccer player, and fisherman you are. And, even more, of what a great person you are becoming. This book is dedicated to you, and so am I.

This book would not have happened were it not for the courage of the Trebing family in opening their lives to the constant presence of a reporter. Thanks especially to Katie Trebing, a little girl who allowed a reporter to play Zingo Bingo with her in her hospital room during her bone marrow procedure and to join her family at numerous medical appointments and family events.

The Trebings participated in this story because they want to see a cure for diseases like Diamond Blackfan anemia so people won't have to make such difficult choices. They want to see people give blood to help those who need it. And their belief in the medical miracle that formed their family of five and healed Katie led them to let others see what it's like to be ordinary people faced with an extraordinary choice.